Healing Walks for Hard Times

Healing Walks for Hard Times

Quiet Your Mind, Strengthen Your Body, and Get Your Life Back

CAROLYN SCOTT KORTGE

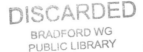

TRUMPETER
Boston & London
2010

Trumpeter Books
An imprint of Shambhala Publications, Inc.
Horticultural Hall
300 Massachusetts Avenue
Boston, Massachusetts 02115
www.shambhala.com

9 8 7 6 5 4 3 2 1

First edition
Printed in the United States of America

♾ This edition is printed on acid-free paper that meets the
American National Standards Institute Z39.48 Standard.
♻ This book was printed on 30% postconsumer recycled paper.
For more information please visit www.shambhala.com.

Distributed in the United States by Random House, Inc., and
in Canada by Random House of Canada Ltd

Interior design and composition: Greta D. Sibley & Associates

Library of Congress Cataloging-in-Publication Data

Kortge, Carolyn Scott.
Healing walks for hard times: quiet your mind, strengthen your body,
and get your life back / Carolyn Scott Kortge.
p.   cm.
Includes bibliographical references and index.
ISBN 978-1-59030-740-3 (pbk.: alk. paper)
1. Walking—Health aspects. 2. Stress (Physiology)—Health aspects.
3. Mental healing. 4. Comtemplation. I. Title.
RA781.65.K66 2010
613.7'176—dc22
2010008310

For Dean,
So lucky to be loving you

Contents

Introduction

Walking is man's best medicine.

—Hippocrates

When the alarm went off at 5 AM, I was waiting for it. Fear had roused me already. I rolled to my side and reached out to silence the buzzer on my bedside table. Slowly, I pulled up into a reluctant hunch at the edge of the bed. The countdown had begun. Two hours to surgery. Two hours to prepare. Two hours to worry and fret. Instinctively, my shoulders pulled forward in a protective reflex. I wrapped my arms across my chest and lingered amid my fears.

How would my body feel to me the next time I woke up? How would it look? How would it be changed by the breast cancer diagnosis that had spilled a chilling terror into my days? A swirl of "what-ifs" and "whys" gripped my mind. I knew what I had to do next. Still, it took a deep breath and a dose of determination to get me out for a walk. It wasn't simply habit that moved me. It was willful effort—an intentional pursuit of mental calmness.

The cool air of a May morning awakened my senses as I turned onto a neighborhood street. My husband fell into step at my side in silence. The rhythm of his footsteps steadied me as we settled into the hush of a new day. Soon, the words of a familiar chant began to roll through my head. *I am walk-ing. I am breath-ing. I am walk-ing. I am breath-ing,* I repeated mentally. The words matched the rhythm of my steps and breath, creating a steady, four-beat cadence.

Over and over, the phrase cycled through my mind. When fears intruded on the phrase, I started over again. *I am walk-ing. I am breath-ing.* The pattern was soothing. It silenced uncertainties that tumbled through my thoughts and quieted the fears that pursued me as I prepared for surgery. Earlier in my life, I'd used these words to block the self-doubt that tripped me up in athletic competition. They reminded me to breathe and to move. Fresh air in; stale air out. Nothing else right now.

On this day, I needed the words as a shield against panic. For two weeks, I had been grappling with the questions a crisis unleashes. Why did this happen to me? What should I do next? What did I do to deserve this? Over and over. Around and around. The questions taunted me. The struggle is familiar to everyone who has been leveled by a life-changing event or diagnosis. Nothing will ever be quite the same again. In such times, we grope for something familiar to provide reassurance, stability, and a respite from the storm. Sometimes it's a friend or family member. Sometimes music. Sometimes prayer or an uplifting poem.

For me, reassurance stretched along the sidewalks of my neighborhood. I'd been walking them for years. Once these streets had presented a training challenge as I discovered an athlete hidden inside me. Back then, I measured off a mile and bought a stopwatch to clock my walking pace. The surprising thrill of endorphins and physical exertion led me to learn racewalking techniques. At age forty-six, I entered my first track meet.

Athletic competition was an exhilarating experience. It opened a new outlet for my competitive spirit and rewarded me with national medals. But my greatest achievement as an athlete was learning to heal the philosophical fragmentation of body, mind, and spirit that had governed my approach to life. Success in competition demanded a unified effort—body, mind, and spirit working as one. By focusing on breath, or on positive words, I learned to control the erratic distractions of my active mind. I discovered the power, and the joy, in alignment—in all of me working together toward a shared goal. I felt whole. When I stopped competing as a racewalker, I settled back into fitness walking and used the tools of athletic competition to make my steps an active meditation. *The Spirited Walker: Fitness Walking for Clarity, Balance, and Spiritual Connection,* which I wrote a few years ago, shares my journey from walking competition to walking meditation.

A cancer diagnosis two years after publication of that book catapulted me into a new kind of competition—competition with a life-threatening disease. Who could have imagined that the skills of athletic competition would emerge as a resource now? My training as a racewalker left a lifetime impact. It taught me to walk through my fears. It gave me the experience of pushing past the doubts that gripped my spirit when I felt myself losing face, or speed, or focus in a race. It taught me that movement opens pathways for the release of tension and fear.

Perhaps that experience made it easier for me to fight the impulse to withdraw on the morning of my surgery. Still, I assure you that walking was an act of willpower. A conscious choice to stop—even for a few seconds at a time—the uncertainty and terror that dominated my emotions. Before surgical preparations began, I wanted to feel myself moving on a path where I felt safe. At a time when so many issues in my life seemed out of my control, walking reaffirmed the choices I still had. I walked as a personal statement of faith, a physical demonstration of my intention to keep moving. Keep taking steps. Keep living here and now.

Mapping a Healing Journey

When you are facing an enormous personal challenge, taking control of something as basic as a walk may seem insignificant. But research suggests that even small acts of control can help you recover from the feeling of hopelessness that often accompanies trauma. Sustained helplessness upsets the body's endocrine system by suppressing immune functions and elevating production of stress hormones. The ability to find even a small area of control triggers healing, both in the spirit and in the chemicals that regulate the body.

The walk I took before surgery for breast cancer was my way of maintaining some small sense of control. I couldn't control the outcome of a cancer diagnosis, but I *could* control the impulse to stay in bed and tremble. Throughout chemotherapy and radiation, I walked. Friends and family accompanied me at times, lending support to steps that informed my cells I was not giving up. Cancer changed the course of my walks as I moved through transitions from victim to patient to survivor—and then, eventually, to victor, bringing my experience and my restored health to a new walking goal. Two years after my diagnosis, the medical center where I was treated invited me to teach a walking clinic for cancer patients and supporters. We met weekly for a month in the parking lot and practiced taking control of little things— like breathing and self-talk. Week by week, we explored a path of healing together.

The profound relief experienced by people in stress—whether from illness, family crisis, depression, professional burnout, or an argument with a friend—emerged in those classes as the real rewards of mindful walking. Focusing techniques I had used in meditation and in athletic performance became elements of healing on walks that restore balance and momentum.

"This class was exactly what I needed at this time," a participant told me at the end of the four-week program. "I left each class feeling energized, happy, confident, and contented. And it lasts."

In recent years, I have had opportunities to share these ideas in workshops across the United States. At medical centers, wellness conferences, fitness resorts, and healing retreats, I meet people who want movement in their lives. They long to clear a path through the mental fog that accompanies stressful situations. They know they "should" be exercising, but they lack a clear direction. From them I have learned that it takes more than research data or nagging family members to keep an exercise program going when life is in upheaval. *It takes compassion and a plan.* This book responds to that need.

Healing Walks for Hard Times delivers an eight-week guided walking program that leads you to renewed energy and to healing. The weekly Walking Well plan advances chapter by chapter with a progressive series of mental and physical steps that help you get back on track with your life, at your own pace.

In the beginning, each walk is a choice that must be made in the mind. It isn't an easy choice when you're struggling with issues that deplete body, energy, spirit, or faith. This program simplifies the decision to move. Follow the guidelines and you are on your way. Each week you will be taking steps that help you regain your footing. The steps you take are not simply physical. Movement begins in the mind . . . with the will to move.

If you're a nonexerciser whose interest in fitness has been stimulated by an event that jarred your life, be understanding as you launch this new activity. Remember, it's never too late to start moving. Now it's time to focus forward, rather than looking back to criticize past patterns.

If you were once a regular exerciser but now can't seem to find the energy to push beyond the mire of decisions and doubts that hard times produce, take a breath and let go of self-judgment.

If you're a former athlete who has lost momentum due to physical or emotional difficulties, be considerate as you get back on your feet. Hard times are hard times. We all need to sit down and stop occasionally. It's OK. Now you're ready to stand up and move forward again. Slowly and sensibly. Gently, with kindness and understanding.

This book is for all of you.

Healing Walks for Hard Times

Starting Out

When You Walk through a Storm, Keep Your Feet on the Ground

*K*eep your feet on the ground," we tell ourselves when hard times shake the foundations that support us. "One step at a time," caring friends urge when disappointment, disaster, or disease plunge life into turmoil. It's sound advice and familiar. References to walking are so deeply embedded in our language they have become clichés. The words have power because they reflect our experience. We know how it feels to get knocked off balance, and what it means to get back on our feet. The phrases remind us that movement is both external and internal—move the body and you move the spirit.

In times of upheaval and stress, the familiar phrases offer more than reassurance; they deliver a prescription for recovery. Walking is a profound tool of healing. When spirits droop and footsteps falter, walking awakens the healing powers of the human spirit, literally, with chemicals that change the way you feel. Each step launches a chain reaction of healing that's both physical and mental. Whether the wound is physical, emotional, professional, or spiritual, a walk can ease the grip of hard times, delivering an antidote to despair. But each step requires an act of faith.

You've taken the first step already by picking up this book. *Healing Walks for Hard Times* outlines a path of healing that makes getting your feet on the ground as natural as taking a walk. It simplifies the process with a progressive eight-week walking program that guides your steps. As you travel through the following chapters, you'll discover that healing is gradual. Often the physical act of walking mirrors the internal movement that accompanies healing. With each walk, you begin to move ahead in a life that has been shaken.

Unlike most walking books, this one does not dwell on walking for physical fitness or health or weight loss. The focus here is on *walks that heal*—walks that help you bridge the chasm from helplessness to healing—from victim to survivor.

In the following pages, you will meet people like you—people from many backgrounds, lifestyles, and areas, who have encountered hard times and found their way through the turmoil on a walking path. Let their experiences encourage and inspire your own healing journey. It is a journey of acceptance. It begins with choosing to take the first step.

After the death of his twenty-one-year-old son, Terry Gray took the first step simply because Josie needed a walk. She whined at the door until the grieving father picked up a leash and fell into step with the Black Mouth Cur that his son had adopted as a pup. Three or four times a day, the dog prodded Terry from the torpor of his grief and led him on walks that anchored his days in reality and set a pattern of recovery.

A cancer diagnosis propelled Carrie Wells to buy her first pair of walking shoes and sign up for a benefit walk. She traveled from victim to survivor on a path that made her part of a movement rather than an isolated victim fighting her fears alone.

You can do it, too. Some hard times are physical, arising from illness, accidents, or age. Some are emotional. Some are spiritual.

Just as there are many kinds of hard times, there are many forms of healing. Healing may be an emotional passage that carries you to an understanding of the difference between "cured" and "healed." Where cure is not a possibility, you can still find meaning in each day and value in your life. Step by step, the reassuring momentum of walking can restore direction when your life has been thrown off course.

Walking awakens the profound healing power of the human spirit and carries it into each cell with chemicals that change the way you feel.

We are all aware of the benefits of walking for fitness and physical health. The Side Steps section of this chapter highlights some of the significant findings regarding walking and physical health. The studies build a convincing case for regular exercise, and can provide start-up impetus for a walking program. But in hard times, you may find that you need more than research to sustain commitment and momentum. Statistics fall by the wayside when you are reeling from an encounter with disease, grief, disaster, divorce, depression, accident, or post-traumatic stress—any life-changing event. Even less dramatic losses can deliver a stunning blow. Job loss, a break-in at home, an unjust accusation—all can leave you feeling helpless and hopeless. You long for direction and guidance—a steady hand to lead you through the darkness. *Healing Walks for Hard Times* extends that hand with a personal map to recovery and well-being.

"Solvitur ambulando," promises a Latin phrase attributed to St. Augustine. "It is solved by walking." The truth of Augustine's endorsement remains as valid today as it was in the fourth century. Not everything, of course, is solved by walking. But a good deal is. And if it isn't solved, it is reorganized, refreshed, or revitalized so that new responses are possible. Walking changes perspective. It offers a path that moves us forward, literally and figuratively.

"It is solved by walking."

Turning Your Walks into a Healing Journey

Day by day, step by step, walking sets the body's healing circuitry in motion. Like most prescriptions, walking is most effective when you take it consistently. If you are taking other medicines, you know the importance of regularity. It is the same with exercise. Perhaps it will help you maintain a regular walking program if you think of it as a prescription you need to take daily. The body needs exercise to function optimally. The spirit needs it to renew vitality and zest for life.

In the next eight chapters, you'll be introduced to mental and physical skills that lay the groundwork for healing. If you have participated in athletics at some point in your life, you may recognize many of these skills. If you have listened to relaxation tapes or attended meditation groups, you, too, will be familiar with the mental tools that transform walking into a healing journey. Bringing them into your walks compounds the benefits of your steps. In the weeks ahead, you'll experiment with walks that integrate mental skills used by athletes and by meditators—breath awareness, positive mantras, affirmation, self-talk, and visual imagery. Walking becomes more than physical exercise; it becomes a form of stress release and healing that supports medical treatment and emotional recovery. You boost energy with better breathing, release endorphins that make life brighter, and stimulate enhanced immune functions.

As you learn to put aside the swirl of worry and stress that floods your thoughts in times of upheaval, you'll discover new ways of seeing, hearing, moving, and connecting to yourself and to the world around you. Your walks provide an active meditation that aligns body, mind, and spirit. You'll also learn to engage the power of "cognitive override," a skill that researchers call the secret to a lasting exercise program. It means, simply, using your intellectual strength to make decisions that are in your best interest, even when your spirit feels low. You already use cognitive override in daily life, although you probably don't call it that. Cognitive override is what gets you up in the morning when the alarm goes off. It's the internal control that fights temptation when you feel like eating the whole carton of ice cream. It is the wisdom to make a good choice.

Cognitive override is a concept that lies at the core of recovery when life knocks you down. It's the tool that helps you get back on your feet—a key to the resiliency that identifies a survivor. Each time you take a walk, you demonstrate your intention to survive. You may not know where life will lead you next, or what path you'll travel, but you do know how to take one step at a time. That's how healing begins. Each step reawakens the will to live and the strength to move on.

Tune In

As you integrate mindfulness into your walks, I urge you to turn off your music or cell phone. When you walk in silence, you allow yourself to heal from the inside out. You reconnect with your own inner strength and wisdom. You also connect with the world around you. In nature, in the weather, in the people sharing the sidewalks, you become aware of the resiliency of life and the cycles of the seasons. Make a practice of spending a portion of each walk in silence.

Nothing changes if nothing changes.

When walking with another person, negotiate for a period of silence. It may feel awkward at first. It may be unfamiliar. But if you want something to change in your life, you have to be willing to try something different. As one of my favorite aphorisms says: "Nothing changes if nothing changes!" Initiate the change by taking time to connect with yourself.

After I stopped training as a competitive racewalker and slowed my pace, my husband asked to join me on my morning walks. I worried privately that his presence would intrude on the focused silence I had come to value. Gently, I proposed a strategy: What if we talked for ten or fifteen minutes, sharing plans for the day as we warmed up? Then, we could settle into silence for the rest of our neighborhood loop. In a few days, we found a comfortable pattern. Work schedules, chores, and weekend plans held our focus as we set out. Gradually, conversation drifted aside, and we walked side by side with the rhythm of our steps affirming a companionship that didn't depend on talk. Our walks brought a closeness I hadn't expected—a bond shaped by our footsteps. The change I'd feared became a change for the better.

Reach Out

There will be days when you'll need help in order to sustain a pattern of healthy walks. Disruptions or depression may cloud your resolve. This guided walking program provides one form of help by supplying a format that simplifies each step. You may also find that willpower, cognitive override, or a walking partner deliver added backup for your commitment to healing walks.

So often, the people in our lives want to be helpful in times of difficulty, but they don't know what to do. Ask them to assist you by walking at your side, in silence and support. No need for endless repetition of the problems in your life. Just move forward together. Walks that enable you to connect with friends or family can be helpful for you, and also for those who care about you. Crises are rarely one-person events. Be it disease, disaster, or the death of a loved one, the blow reverberates far beyond the person first in line. Family members, office colleagues, church associates, friends all share the loss of stability that crisis creates. In recent years a new term—co-survivor—has appeared to acknowledge the role of those who journey through a trauma at the side of someone else. They become "survivors," too.

Some people contend that "survivorship" begins the moment disaster strikes. If you are alive right now, you're a survivor, they say. In the end, I think that it's a change of attitude, as much as anything, that defines a survivor. Life can't be taken for granted anymore. Thich Nhat Hanh, a Vietnamese Buddhist monk and author, spoke from his vantage point as a survivor of the Vietnam

War when he wrote the morning prayer with which he greets the day:

> Waking up this morning, I smile; twenty-four brand new hours before me. I vow to live fully in each moment, and to look at all beings with eyes of compassion.[1]

It is a prayer that challenges us to live with the mindfulness of a survivor—aware and appreciative. It reminds us that compassion includes compassion toward ourselves. One day, one step at a time.

The Next Step

How do you begin a walking program when your body is physically, emotionally, and spiritually depleted? How do you get back on your feet when life has knocked you to your knees? With gentleness. With guidance. With compassion. Let this walking program coach you. Each of the next eight chapters concludes with a Walking Well section where you'll find guidelines for walks at three different levels of physical fitness, energy, and emotional strength.

Consider your daily schedule and medical condition when you decide how much time you can set aside for a walk. Begin where you are and build up. Walk to the mailbox and back instead of waiting for someone else to bring in the mail. Go to the end of the block and back. There are no rules about the goals you set. Each week you'll get a chance to revise and reassess. Be willing to experiment with new thoughts and new patterns of exercise as you follow weekly outlines that simplify the process of building healthy habits. Each week builds on the previous week, so your endurance and skills increase as you move through the book.

No matter which level you select as a starting point, the weeks ahead will introduce you to mindful focusing techniques that restore balance and wholeness. You'll probably discover that you enjoy some of the focusing tools more than others. That's normal.

Some exercises may seem repetitious. That's intentional. Many techniques build on previous exercises, in a process I think of as adding "layers." Each layer expands or varies the focus to give you more ways to still the turmoil of a busy brain. The more options you explore, the more resources you'll have when you encounter resistance to just getting out the door.

There's no need to read the entire book before taking the first walk. In fact, I suggest you move ahead one week at a time, following the walks for that week. Remember that restored health and well-being don't happen with a snap of the finger. Neither do habits. They emerge as a result of repetition.

Choose a Course

To make walking fit easily into your routine, find a place to walk that is near your home or work. Peaceful parks are wonderful but not always convenient. The sidewalks or lanes of your neighborhood probably are fine. If you walk the same route, you'll know after a few days how many minutes it takes you to get to the corner, or to the mailbox, where you turn around. Then you can give full attention to the mindfulness techniques introduced in every chapter.

When weather conditions make the outdoors unpleasant, find a shopping mall, athletic club, or covered walkway where you can keep moving. Many malls open early to give walkers an exercise route that's warm, dry, and clear of shoppers. Treadmills offer a convenient indoor alternative. Research reveals that treadmill walkers achieve the same stress release and energy benefits as outdoor walkers. Just remember to turn off the television some of the time you are on the treadmill. The goal of Walking Well is to "zone in" not to "zone out." By practicing awareness and mindfulness, you strengthen inner resources.

Gear Up

Comfortable, supportive walking shoes are the most important gear for this program. If you don't already have these, find an athletic store that specializes in running and walking shoes. That's where you'll encounter sales representatives who have been trained to fit athletic shoes. Walk around with the shoes on before you buy them to be sure you have a good fit. A good shoe helps prevent problems down the road. And so does a *new* shoe.

Most walking shoes lose adequate cushioning and support after 300 to 500 miles, depending on individual weight and stride. That may sound like a lot of miles, but if you walk at a moderate pace for twenty minutes, six days a week, you'll log almost 400 miles in a year. Bump it up to thirty minutes, six times a week, and you'll cover 500 miles a year. Time for new shoes!

Moisture-wicking socks are another smart investment for walkers. They reduce the risk of blisters that are more common with all-cotton or all-wool socks. Proper socks and shoes help reduce discomfort that can undermine your good intentions about exercise.

A digital sports watch is one of my favorite nonessential walking accessories. It helps to have a dial that is easy to read when you want to time your walks. Without a watch to keep you honest, it's easy to fool yourself about how long you've been moving. If you don't have a digital watch and don't want to invest in one, a portable kitchen timer is a fine alternative. Set it for five minutes, stick it in your pocket, and you are ready to go.

Get Ready, Get Set

You probably have a fairly clear idea of how far or how long you are able to walk comfortably right now. As you start this walking program, begin at the low end of your fitness level and expand as you feel ready. If you try one level and discover you want more exercise, add an additional block to your distance. If you're having a difficult week and energy is low, choose walks from the Stepping Out level. It's important to let yourself modify your activity rather than give up and abandon the program completely. Any amount of walking will help restore connection of body, mind, and spirit. The descriptions below will help you select a starting goal for your own healing walks.

Any amount of walking will help restore connection of body, mind, and spirit. Modify your goals rather than abandon the program completely.

If you have physical limits due to injury or medications, please check with medical advisors before beginning a walking program. If you've been working with a physical therapist or exercise physiologist in recovering from injury or surgery, consult that person regarding appropriate goals for your present condition. If you are experiencing difficulty with balance, you may need to walk with the assistance of a cane, a walker, or a supportive friend. Diabetes, obesity, back surgeries, and some chemotherapy drugs can impair feeling in the feet, making walkers unsteady. You need not let these obstacles stop you completely. Instead, treat yourself gently by accepting support that will assist you in succeeding. You're embarking on a path of healing that begins with compassion toward yourself.

STEPPING OUT—START-UP LEVEL: *Ten-Minute Walks, Six Days a Week*

If you haven't been exercising at all or if you have health challenges that make walking difficult, begin prudently and respectfully. The length of each walk is not as important as your consistency in establishing a habit that makes you stronger, less stressed, and more resilient. A reasonable goal for the first week might be a ten-minute walk on six days. If that's more than you feel comfortable doing, start with a five-minute walk twice a day. If you want to walk seven days, it's fine. At this level of exercise, your body does not need a day of recovery.

Make the routine easy by heading out the door and walking for five minutes. Turn around and walk back. That's it—ten minutes of exercise. It doesn't matter how *far* you go. What matters is *that* you go. Walk the length of the parking lot and back and you'll fit exercise into a trip to the grocery store. The second week, you might try adding just one minute to the time you walk before turning around, lengthening the walk by a total of two minutes. Add two minutes each week to your walks, and you'll be up to twenty-four minutes per walk by the end of this eight-week program. Sustain the pattern for three more weeks and you'll reach thirty minutes per walk. That's a 300 percent increase in walking time in just three months!

MID-STRIDE—MODERATE LEVEL: *Twenty-Minute Walks, Six Days a Week*

Maybe you haven't been exercising much recently but you do not have physical limits that make walking difficult. Choose a goal that pushes you to get moving most days of the week. A reasonable starting goal would be to walk for twenty minutes, six days a week. After a week or two at this starting level, you may be ready to increase the length of your walks by three to four minutes. Or you might try a thirty-minute walk once a week.

If you experience no pain when you lengthen your walks, you may find that by week four, you are ready to walk three days for twenty minutes and three days for thirty minutes. That's a 25 percent increase in walking time in one month. By the end of the program, you may be ready for thirty minutes daily, a level that meets the Surgeon General's recommendation for health maintenance. You will have added a full hour of walking time weekly and increased both physical and emotional strength.

STRONG AND STEADY—FIT AND ACTIVE LEVEL: *Thirty-Minute Walks, Six Days a Week*

If you are a former exerciser whose fitness routines have been disrupted by life events, you know how good it feels to move regularly. But physical or emotional difficulties can sideline even the most enthusiastic walker. Now you're ready to reestablish a pattern that gets you moving again with a combination of physical activity and mental tools that encourage healing. If you are physically ready, you may want to start with thirty-minute walks, six days a week.

Outlines at this level will provide opportunities to increase distance or pace as you experiment with being present and mindful. If you are a seasoned walker, it may not be distance goals that you need from this program. Instead, you may be seeking the peace of mind that can be provided by melding meditation techniques with your steps. If that's the case for you, walk as far and as often as is your custom and put your focus on making changes in the mental awareness you bring to your exercise. Learn to use your breathing, posture, and self-talk to support healing of spirit, or to restore trust in life.

Moving On

The map is here; your role is to take the next steps. Make modifications, when necessary, so that you keep moving at a time or pace you can maintain. Be flexible. If you can't walk at the time or day you planned, choose another time. Put on your raincoat or knit cap when weather is a challenge. You already know that unexpected things happen in life. Healing comes with acknowledging the disruption and moving on, finding an alternative. Even short walks boost energy levels and allow you to clear your mind.

Make History

Research indicates that people who keep exercise logs have greater success in sticking with a new activity. By writing down goals and recording your walks, you create a reward system that keeps you involved and motivated. Why not start now? In the appendix of this book, you'll find Walking Logs for each week of this program. The logs look like this:

Week One

Date: __May 15–22__

Walk Days	Walk Time		Silent Segment	Health and Fitness Notes	Nature Notes, Comments, Appreciation
Sun.	Goal	20 min.	10 min.	No pain in knee! Moderate energy.	Crisp morning, cool, fresh air. Saw two housefinches on feeder. Love my new shoes.
	Done	23 min.	23 min.		
Tues.	Goal	20 min.	15 min.	Challeng-ing to breathe in and out nose.	Vibrant sunset colors in sky this evening. New marigolds plant=ed at corner house. Calm and peaceful.
	Done	25 min.	10 min.		
Wed.	Goal	20 min.	10 min.	A bit tired to-day. Up too late last night.	Windy, smell of mown grass in air. Cool breeze on skin helped wake me up!
	Done	15 min.	10 min.		

Weekly logs give you a place to write and reflect on your goals. Put the starting date for the week at the top of the log. Then, decide which days you will walk. Make it your goal to walk six days a week with an option for seven days if you feel like it. Next, write how long you commit to walk—ten minutes, twenty minutes, and so on—in the space that asks for Walk Time. How many minutes will you spend in silence during that walk? Write that number in the appropriate space. As you follow the eight-week Walking Well program, record how much time you actually walk each day. How many minutes in silence? Add comments that personalize your experience. How was your energy? How did your body feel as you walked? What caught your attention? Did you notice something you hadn't been aware of before, either in nature or in yourself? The process of recording observations on a log sharpens your awareness and helps you stay present on each walk.

You might also find it helpful to mark your walk schedule on your calendar, or on a sticky note that you can post on the refrigerator door. This is an agreement with yourself.

The logs are grouped together in the appendix so that you can easily see your progress from week to week. If you don't feel comfortable writing in this book, or if you want to continue keeping a log beyond the eight-week program, use these pages as a template and make copies for an ongoing record of distance, time, and discoveries that emerge from each walk. You can also log on to www.walksthatheal.com and print out log sheets as you need them.

Now it's time to move on. The next chapter leads you on your first walk. It may take a few days, or a few weeks, for you to discover the delight that lies beneath the discipline of a consistent walking program. Keep it up for eight weeks of walking and you'll create a healing habit. Consistency allows you to feel your progress. It enables you to experience the healing that walking delivers for body and soul.

SIDE STEPS: *Walking and Wellness*

Walking brings impressive rewards in stress release, relief from depression, enhanced bone strength, reduced risk of cancer, diabetes, stroke, and heart disease, and improved energy and mood. If you're not convinced, these research findings give an overview of the healing powers of walking.

HEART DISEASE

Brisk walking three hours a week (a pace of 3.5 to 4 miles per hour, thirty minutes a day) cut heart disease risk in women by up to 40 percent in a study of 72,000 female nurses aged forty to sixty-five, in the long-term Nurses' Health Study at Harvard. *New England Journal of Medicine,* August 1999

DEPRESSION

Researchers at Duke University Medical Center found that a brisk thirty-minute walk or jog around a track three times a week was just as effective as antidepressant medication in relieving the symptoms of major depression. *Archives of Internal Medicine*, 1999

CHOLESTEROL

Women who walked three days a week for ten weeks significantly increased levels of beneficial high-density lipoprotein cholesterol (HDL) and decreased triglyceride levels. *Journals of Gerontology*, 2002

OSTEOPOROSIS

A study of 1,000 women and 700 men found that walking protects the bone density of the hips and bone mass in the spine. *American Journal of Epidemiology*, 1995

BREAST CANCER

The Nurses' Health Study found a reduction in breast cancer risk among 122,000 participants who walked or did more vigorous exercise for seven or more hours per week compared with those who exercised one hour or less. *Archives of Internal Medicine*, 1999

Even short walks help. Women who walked briskly for 1.25 to 2.5 hours a week reduced breast cancer risk by 18 percent. *Journal of American Medicine*, 2003

DIABETES

In a four-month study of patients with type-2 diabetes, those who walked for forty-five to sixty minutes, three times a week, improved blood pressure levels and lipid metabolism over patients who did not exercise. *Diabetes Research and Clinical Practice*, January 2006

The National Institutes of Health's Diabetes in March program demonstrated that walking, combined with diet, does more to ward off diabetes than the diabetes-prevention drug Metformin. *Washington Post*, October 1, 2002

MENTAL CLARITY AND PROBLEM SOLVING

Researchers at Ohio State University tested volunteers' ability to fire off words that start with a particular letter. After a ten-week exercise program, participants were retested. The result: more words. A year later, only the ones who continued the exercise regimen retained their "enhanced cognitive function." *Newsweek,* September 27, 2004

IMMUNE SYSTEM FUNCTIONS

Regular moderate exercise not only helps your immune system fight off simple bacterial and viral infections, it also may actually decrease the incidence of illnesses such as heart disease, osteoporosis, and cancer. Physical activity may help by flushing bacteria out from the lungs (thus decreasing the chance of a cold, flu, or other airborne illness) and may flush out carcinogens (cancer-causing cells) by increasing waste output, such as urine and sweat. *Medline* (www.nlm.nih.gov/medlineplus)

Week One

A Healthy Step

Begin a journey of recovery this week with walks that restore trust in the healing power of your body. Connect with the support of your own posture and with the solid ground beneath your feet. As you take steps that fuse movement and mindfulness, you engage a twofold defense against stress and move forward toward health and well-being.

A walking vacation in Greece sounded like a wonderful holiday to Nola Woodbury. A fit, active woman who had trekked in Nepal, hiked in England, and biked 500 miles across her home state, she didn't question her body's readiness for island hikes. In fact, she trusted the physical focus of the trip to restore a healthy balance in her busy life.

But in Greece, her steps took an unexpected route. As she scrambled over the rocky mountain trails that hikers shared with local goats, a heaviness seeped into her arms. She blamed it on a new daypack and stopped to readjust the straps. The change brought no relief. Step by step, the heaviness pursued her until it settled into a dull ache.

A registered nurse in her early fifties, Nola recognized the signs of potential heart trouble. She brushed the thought aside. *Not me*, she told herself. Nothing in her healthy lifestyle made her a candidate for heart attack. In the remaining days of her trip, she trudged slowly along the trails, falling behind other members of the group. The problem, she insisted, came from her equipment, not her body. It was annoying but not serious, she decided.

Back home, she scheduled a doctor's appointment to check an infected blister from the trek. In passing, she mentioned the ache in her arms that had developed as she hiked. By the time the appointment ended, she had been booked into a hospital bed. Emergency bypass surgery corrected a near-complete blockage of blood flow to the left ventricle of her heart, and sent her home with shaken confidence.

"My life did a topsy-turvy," she says.[1] Gratitude wrestled with fear as her thoughts careened between thankfulness for surviving a close call and concern about what other unknown risks might lie ahead. "It's very vulnerable having your heart opened to the world," she says.

She ventured back into daily life with cautious steps. Walking offered a path of healing, but the first outings demanded a gentle rebuilding of trust—trust in her heart and in her head. She started slowly. At her front door, she set a kitchen timer for five minutes and slipped it into her pocket. With arms folded protectively across her chest, she walked down the driveway to the street. When the timer sounded the end of five minutes, she turned around and headed back. Five minutes out. Five minutes back. A short walk but a big step in rebuilding strength and confidence. Twice a day she repeated the journey until gradually she began to trust her heart again.

As she felt stronger, she inched the timer forward, one minute at a time, until eventually she reached a total of twenty minutes twice a day. Then she unfolded her arms and let them swing at her sides. In the rhythm of her movement, she heard the words of a familiar hymn: *God walks beside me, and guides my way, through every moment of every day.* As she walked, she sang the words silently, creating a moving meditation that restored physical and spiritual strength. She replaced thoughts of uncertainty and fear about her heart, her fitness, her future, with a reassuring song.

When we can stop stress-producing thoughts, even for a few minutes, we give the body a moment of peace. It is in these intervals of tranquility that the body experiences an opportunity to heal. When freed of the hovering presence of stress, our bodies register physical and emotional changes that restore healthy functions. The spirit mends as well, which is why people feel increased energy and optimism after a good walk.

"I feel confident in my body now," she reported eighteen months after heart surgery. "I realize we need to be thankful for our bodies and for our ability to move around in the world because it can so quickly be taken from us."

As Nola became comfortable and safe in her body once again, the "change of heart" she experienced extended beyond physical recovery. With new awareness of life's fragility, she decided to pursue a dream. From nursing she moved into theology, becoming an ordained Unity Church minister with a position of leadership in her community church. Her response to a life-threatening health condition is not unusual. Many people find that recovery includes a review of priorities for their lives.

"When hit by a life disrupting change, you will never be the same again. You will emerge either stronger or weaker, either better or bitter. You have within you the ability to determine which way it will be for you,"[2] says Al Siebert, author of *The Resiliency Advantage*. Movement that is physical—walking, jogging, swimming, dancing—helps the body prepare for resiliency by enhancing circulation and energy, which in turn reduces stress. On the symbolic level, it helps us get unstuck.

Cellular Alchemy

Science confirms that exercise activates biochemical changes that bring vitality to the cells. It's not really a mystery why that happens. Movement increases air flow into the lungs. At the same time, the heart beats faster and circulation speeds up. Oxygen pulses into the blood and is carried through the body to nourish the cells. Fresh energy in and waste products out. It is how the body is designed to work.

Hard times disrupt these vital biological processes. Disease or injury may limit your physical ability to move in ways you moved in the past. They may breed fear or distrust of your body. You feel vulnerable and unsafe in your own skin. Lack of sleep, increased anxiety, loss of exercise, and poor eating patterns compound the physical impact of upheaval. Some crises plunge us headfirst into problem solving and a mental quest for answers. Gathering information and options is an essential step in recovery, but it, too, tends to distance the body, pushing physical needs aside as mental uncertainties command full attention. If sustained too long, this separation of mind and body leads to abuse of the physical systems that sustain a healthy life.

Chemically, the body responds to worries or difficulties by producing stress hormones—cortisol, epinephrine, and norepinephrine. Extended exposure to stress keeps the body in a constant state of defense with no time for recovery. It doesn't take a lot of time or fancy equipment to restore your body's natural chemistry. Walking can tip the scales toward healing by stimulating the release of chemicals such as serotonin, dopamine, and endorphins—neuropeptides that reduce stress and promote relaxation.

Movement activates your body's innate healing processes and you begin to rebuild the cooperative connection of mind and body that is crucial to well-being. Even a short walk gets the juices flowing. With just ten minutes of brisk walking you significantly increase mental alertness, reduce anxiety, and elevate mood. In hard times, you may find that simply walking up and down a hallway leads to profound improvements in mental resourcefulness. Movement gets you back on your feet, reestablishing balance and wholeness.

Ten minutes of brisk walking can increase mental alertness, reduce anxiety, and improve mood.

Adding mindfulness to a walk takes healing a step further. The rhythmic movement of walking by itself is relaxing for the body. That is part of the reason it elevates mood and decreases anxiety. But when mindfulness is combined with rhythmic movement, the chemical changes occur more quickly. Research cardiologist Herbert Benson discovered that walkers who focus on a simple word as they walk reach a state of relaxation faster than walkers who let their minds wander. Benson asked a group of research participants to walk while mentally thinking the words *In* and *Out* with each breath. Nothing more. Just repeat those two words: *In, Out, In, Out.* He instructed another group to focus on steps, mentally thinking *Left, Right, Left, Right,* as they put each foot on the ground. Results for both groups revealed significantly faster stress release than in walkers who used no mental focus.[3] Nola achieved the same result, increasing the healing power of her steps when her mind focused on the words of a familiar hymn.

Why was that? For most of us, an unfocused mind is a loose cannon. Sometimes that can be very creative, but more often, our thoughts crash aimlessly through memories and fears, unleashing a barrage of problems and unfinished business. The brain stirs up doubt and guilt and endless "why me's" as it careens from past to future and back again. This is actually the brain's job—to remember and plan and organize. It is very useful to have an active mind. I'm grateful for my hard-working mind. It serves me well much of the time. But even the brain benefits from a break now and then. Because I appreciate the resourcefulness of my brain, I've learned to calm it with gentleness rather than reprimands. When I catch my thoughts plowing through fears and doubts or unanswered questions as I walk, I've developed the habit of responding politely but firmly. *Thank you,* I say to my overactive mental director. *Thank you, but not now. Right now, I am here and I am walking.* Then I return to awareness of my breath or my footsteps. It's a practice that allows me to acknowledge my lively thought processes and then choose to redirect my focus. It's a choice I make over and over as thoughts reappear. I make it because I have experienced the calming benefits of stopping the spin from time to time.

Scottish walker and writer Rory Stewart discovered the meditative side of walking when he took two years off from his work as a British diplomat and set out in 2000 to walk from Turkey to Bangladesh. A 6,000-mile journey, mostly alone and on foot, carried Rory through Pakistan, India, Nepal, and Afghanistan, and led him to connection with himself, as well as with the people he met and stayed with on the path.

"In the center of Nepal, I began to count my breaths and my steps, and to recite phrases to myself, pushing thoughts away," he writes in *The Places in Between,* a book about his trek. "This is the way some people meditate. I could only feel that calm for at most an hour a day. It was, however, a serenity I had not felt before. It was what I valued most about walking."[4]

It is significant that Rory reached that state of serenity not by striving to make his mind blank, but rather by actively guiding his mind. Focus on a word or phrase brings a pause to the automatic flood of stress-provoking thoughts. Healing chemicals are released into the body, transported by the boost in circulation and oxygen that comes with deep breathing and movement. Walking becomes both exercise and meditation. Step by step, body and mind move into harmony to restore balance, stability, and a sense of wholeness.

Healing Steps for Cells and Psyche

Both exercise and meditation reduce the chemical toll that stress places on immune functions and on mental and physical health. Put them together, and you engage a twofold defense against harmful, persistent stress. The Side Steps section in this chapter highlights research confirming the benefit of exercise and meditation on stress and the immune system. The key is simply to move. There are no *wrong* ways to make walking a part of your daily life. Rather, there are *many* ways to create and sustain a healthy, healing walking schedule. Learn to incorporate mindfulness and variety into your walking program and you'll increase pleasure and benefits.

Physical Balance

Balance begins with your feet. As you set out on this walking program, a helpful way to restore the physical and emotional balance you seek in your life is by giving attention to your footsteps. One of the focusing techniques you will practice this week reestablishes connection with your body, starting with your feet. They are the foundation upon which you restore momentum. By noticing the feel of the earth, or the sidewalk, beneath the sole of your shoes, you draw attention to the present, to this moment, this place, and this act of taking a step.

As you move awareness up your body from your feet, you'll discover that posture also reveals the significant relationship of body and spirit. When an emotional crisis collapses the structure of daily life, it's not unusual for the body to collapse as well. Shoulders roll in, the head droops, and we slump into a posture of hopelessness. Rising up in a strong, erect position is a physical act of intention. It signals a readiness to resume forward movement in life—a willingness to face the world again.

Good posture isn't complicated, but it does require surveillance and practice. You may have physical conditions that force compromises in posture. That's OK. Mindfulness begins simply with becoming aware of your body and your posture as you walk. Strive to maintain the most supportive posture possible. It is a practice that assists both physical and mental balance.

- Keep your torso upright, shoulders relaxed and spine erect, to allow expansion of your lungs with each breath.
- To lift the spine, think about gently lengthening the back of your neck.
- If you don't need a cane or walker for stability, keep your arms free and let them swing at your sides. This movement echoes the rhythm of your steps, loosening shoulders and releasing tension.
- Keep your eyes fixed on a point a bit ahead of you on the path. If your head drops forward so that you're looking at your feet, breathing becomes restricted.

- Be aware of your body as you begin each walk so you move in a way that supports good breathing and good balance.

Mental Balance

When life is challenging, we can't avoid grieving what's been lost. You need not deny or ignore the negative elements in life, but you can begin to balance the pain a bit by recognizing what's positive as well. Psychologist Dan Baker calls appreciation "the antidote to fear."[5] It is impossible, he says, to feel appreciation and fear at the same time. With the act of expressing appreciation, focus shifts away from what is missing or what is wrong, and turns to what is still working, what is beautiful, what is good in the world. Even a moment or two of appreciation creates a brief, healing break in the chain of laments that overwhelms us.

It isn't only in hard times that we can benefit from a minute of appreciation. So much of the time, life bombards us with announcements of some new product or experience or relationship that we absolutely must get if we want to be really happy. Media sources pummel us with reminders of what we don't have—enough time, enough money, the right job, the right car, the best cell phone, the whitest teeth, and on and on. Rarely are we urged to focus on the assets we have. By actively seeking things you can appreciate as you walk, you make a profound shift in awareness. You also boost your odds of success in maintaining an exercise routine.

Gratitude, it turns out, is an integral component of health and well-being. People who keep a weekly journal listing five things they appreciated during the week exercise more regularly and feel better about their lives, discovered psychologists Robert Emmons and Michael McCullough.[6] People who keep gratitude lists are also more likely to make progress toward achieving important personal goals. If you want to boost your odds of success in your commitment to daily walks, consider exercising appreciation while you exercise your body. This week's guidelines introduce a mindfulness tool that makes gratitude a regular feature of your walks. Use the weekly logs that accompany the program to record thoughts of appreciation that emerge from your walks.

Appreciation is an exercise in expanding your point of view. As you exercise your sense of gratitude, you may find that you are able to notice your own successes and accomplishments more readily. Gratitude encourages generosity and compassion, researchers say. It's often difficult to have compassion for ourselves in times of despair. We bemoan the loss of energy and strength that we are experiencing. The mind spins out a chorus of judgments and complaints: *I used to be able to walk from home to the library without a problem. Now look at me! I can't even get halfway! What's the use?*

Compassion is the voice inside that can find a balanced point of view. Compassion knows how to confront the inner critic: *Yes, it's different now, but at least I'm moving. I'm taking steps. Not stuck. Not giving up. That's something to feel good about.* It's not always easy, but it's effective in rebuffing anger or helplessness.

A Steady Pace

We've all heard the saying, "Practice makes perfect." I think that's wrong. Practice makes patterns. As you take your first steps on a new walking program this week, I encourage you to practice creating patterns that support health and wholeness for body, mind, and spirit. Repetition helps your mind and body settle into the rhythm of walking and trains your cells to relax as you walk. Guiding your focus with the various mindfulness techniques outlined each week helps you avoid drifting off course mentally into a thicket of worries and fears.

While it's often true that "the first step is the hardest," it's also true that goals are attained one step at a time. The model for success in getting back on your feet with a walking program lies in the lessons of a classic tale—Aesop's fable of the tortoise and the hare. In exercise, as in the story, the best bet for long-term success rests with the slow and steady progress of the tortoise rather than with the hare's erratic energy. In case you've forgotten the details of the fable, the tortoise is offended when the hare mocks his ponderous walking pace, so he challenges the rabbit to a race. The hare leaps to an easy lead and then decides that since he is so far out in front he might as well lie down in the sun and take a nap. The tortoise plods steadily ahead, focused on the goal. Eventually, he passes the sleeping bunny and goes on to claim the victory. Moral of the story: when setting a new exercise goal, go with the tortoise, not the hare.

SIDE STEPS: *Walking and Immune System*

You're probably familiar with the effects of stress on the body's natural defenses. You've battled a cold that settles in when you are working frantically to complete a deadline project. You've felt the surge in your heart rate that accompanies the shrill blast of a smoke detector. You know the churning that knits the stomach into knots when you wait for results of a medical test. What can you do? Stress is an unavoidable aspect of life. But not all stress is equal.

Anything that triggers a sense of danger or discomfort activates the body's "flight or fight" responses. Your body signals its readiness to help you in a crisis by increasing production of chemicals that boost heart rate and alertness. These chemicals are helpful in meeting the short-term stresses of an insect bite, a warning shout, or a Toastmasters' meeting. But when the stressful situation cannot be resolved, immunity begins to suffer from the continued production of cortisol and other stress-related chemicals.

Researchers say the most damaging impact on immune function comes from chronic stressors—conditions that change people's identities or social roles, conditions that seem beyond control and persist a long time. The longer the stress, the greater the suppression of immunity.[7]

Fortunately, you can help rebuild your body's immune system. Both exercise and meditation bring prompt, effective benefits.

HOW EXERCISE HELPS

Brisk walking bolsters many functions of the immune system.

- *Increased white blood cells.* Regular, moderate exercise restores immune system functions by sending antibodies and white blood cells (the body's defense cells) through the body at a quicker rate. When these white blood cells circulate more rapidly, they can detect illnesses earlier.

- *Increased circulation.* Researchers believe an increased rate of circulation may also trigger the release of hormones that identify intruding bacteria or viruses.
- *Reduced germ spread.* In addition, the elevation of body temperature that results from physical activity may inhibit bacterial growth, allowing the body to fight an infection more effectively.[8]
- *Reduced cortisol production.* Moderate exercise has been shown to reduce the secretion of stress-related hormones and give a temporary boost in the production of macrophages, the cells that attack bacteria.

Even relatively low levels of aerobic exercise protect your immune system. The intensity and amount of effort needed to support the immune system is less than that needed to provide cardiovascular conditioning. How much exercise do you need to achieve immune system benefits? Brisk walks of thirty-five minutes, five days a week, reduced sick days almost by half for participants in one study.[9] But shorter walks also help. The key, say researchers, is consistency and moderation. The benefits of exercise on the immune system are temporary and must be maintained by making regular activity a part of daily life.

HOW MEDITATION HELPS

The value of meditation as a tool for combating the damaging effects of excess stress has been demonstrated so often that meditation and relaxation programs are now offered in many medical centers.

- *Reduced muscle tension.* Herbert Benson, MD, is a cardiologist who coined the term "relaxation response" to identify the body's ability to release stress and balance physical responses. Benson found that meditation helped people activate healthy changes in body chemistry including decreases in blood pressure and muscle tension. By reducing muscle tension, meditation helps lessen inflammation, headache, and other types of pain.

- *Reduced anxiety.* Meditation brought positive changes in the brains and immune systems of university students in an eight-week program at the University of Wisconsin–Madison. "Our findings indicate that a short training program in mindfulness meditation has demonstrable effects on brain and immune function," concluded Richard Davidson, PhD, professor of psychology and psychiatry and coresearcher for the study, along with author Jon Kabat-Zinn, PhD.[10]
- *Increased immune function.* Used as a form of stress reduction, meditation is reported to improve immune system health and promote remission in patients with autoimmune disorders. Medical research suggests that three twenty-minute periods of meditation a week are enough to sustain biological changes, including long-term reduction in heart rate, blood pressure, anxiety, and stress-related problems.

When will you find time to meditate? Do it while you walk! People who combine rhythmic exercise such as walking with mindfulness by counting steps or repeating a meaningful word or phrase activate the "relaxation response" more quickly than walkers who let thoughts wander.[11] By integrating meditative techniques into your exercise program, your steps lead to healing and renewal.

Walking opens us up. It feeds us. As we do the work
necessary to shape and reshape our lives . . . we can walk
our way out of "problem" and into "solution."

—Julia Cameron, *The Vein of Gold*

Healing, like walking, is a progressive, step-by-step process. As you set out on this walking program, your very steps begin to rebuild stability and safety in your life. Any jarring event can trigger an emotional imbalance, and the fastest way to get your feet back on the ground emotionally is often to get both feet on the ground literally. Take a walk and you begin to connect with the stability of the earth and with the physical power to move forward.

This week, your feet will lead you on a journey of discovery. By integrating focusing techniques into your walks, you create a moving meditation that releases stress and restores balance. No matter which fitness level you have chosen as a starting point, these walks reinforce resiliency. Each walk builds on the previous walk to enhance physical and emotional strength.

Because it's easier to maintain focus when you give your mind a change of direction from time to time, each walk outline suggests several mindfulness techniques. By rotating focus, you'll be learning to replace stressful thoughts with focusing tools that keep mind and body connected and present. The guidelines include suggested lengths of time to devote to each mindfulness technique as you move through your walk. These times are simply a starting point for you. Use them as an introductory guide and vary them as you wish when you encounter a focus tool that resonates with your current mood.

After you confirm which level you will follow this week, you might find it helpful to jot down a brief outline of your plan for the week and take it along on your walks. That way, when your mind drifts off course, or when emotional fatigue dulls your memory, you can pull the list out of a pocket and bring yourself back to the focusing techniques you are learning this week. Choose to be present, aware of the steps that move you forward.

Some of the longer walks outlined below for the Mid-Stride and Strong and Steady programs include optional Walk, Talk, Listen segments. These warm-up times allow you to customize your walk. Chat with a friend if you want, listen to music if you choose. But maintain silence during the mental focus segments. Even if you are accustomed to walking with music or a cell phone, try something new. Isn't that what you are looking for with this program? A new habit? A new sense of well-being? If it feels awkward at first to walk in silence, be patient. You will find that with practice it becomes quite comforting.

Quick Tips for Good Posture

- Make sure your spine is straight.
- Keep your shoulders relaxed and back.
- Lift your rib cage to open your lungs.
- Keep your head up and level, eyes focused several feet ahead of you.
- Allow your arms to swing freely at your sides, unless using a cane or a walker.

1. PUT YOUR FOOT DOWN

Turn your attention to your feet for this exercise. Feel each foot touch the ground or the surface beneath you. Do you feel the sole of your foot? What is the texture of the surface holding you? Soft? Bumpy? Smooth? Notice as much detail as you can with each step, being aware that you are on solid footing.

As you continue to walk, imagine that each foot is a kind of rocker, like the bottom of a rocking chair. When you take a step, touch the earth first at the back of the rocker, your heel. Then roll forward, to the toes. Each step becomes a smooth forward roll that prolongs your connection with the solid support of the ground. Feel yourself moving easily, smoothly ahead, on rocker feet that caress the earth. Mindful footwork has the benefit of supporting good walking posture and reducing stressful impact on joints. If you want to add a verbal cue, you can mentally say *left, right, left, right,* as you move from foot to foot.

2. BREATHE IN, BREATHE OUT

Bring awareness of breath to your walks and you are practicing a common tool of meditation to quiet the nonstop babble of an active mind. As you walk, mentally coach yourself by saying *In* as you inhale a fresh breath. When you exhale, mentally say *Out* as air flows out of your lungs. The words keep your mind engaged so that you really notice each breath. *In, Out, In, Out.* Maintain a slow, steady rhythm, letting the words guide you to take in a full, deep breath and then let it all out. Probably you'll find that simply saying the words in your mind helps you breathe deeper than usual. This simple exercise quickly moves your focus away from other things swirling through your head. Notice how different this breathing feels from when you are walking and talking with a friend.

3. FOUR-STEP

This exercise takes advantage of the familiar cadence of a march to control the mental spiral of your thoughts. It puts the focus on the rhythm of your steps. Begin by simply counting your foot-steps in your head: *One-two-three-four, One-two-three-four.* Nothing else. Just count the steps. That's all it takes to help the body release stress! Research has shown that walkers who match words with steps release stress more quickly than walkers who let their minds wander.[12] That's because when you think you are relaxing, your mind is likely to be rushing around churning up things to worry about, plan for, or stew over. These are things that wear you out. By counting steps, you break the automatic thought patterns that generate stress.

When your mind wanders, as it will, call it back with *Not now.* Return to the rhythm of the cadence, counting each step—*One-two-three-four, One-two-three-four.* No matter how often your thoughts bound away, bring your focus back to the count. This is moving meditation. You are creating moments of wholeness in which mind and body move together, forming a healthy connection.

4. SAY THANK YOU

I like to end every walk with gratitude. When life is challenging and troubled, it's natural that attention turns to what's wrong. We grumble and complain about our bodies. We focus on trying to fix things or wishing for a miracle. In fact, appreciation is often that miracle. Change the pattern by giving appreciation to body parts that are working fine. Give thanks for your feet that carried you through a walk today. Give thanks for your walking shoes. Give thanks for the sidewalk that provides a smooth place to walk. Give thanks for the willpower that got you moving today. Give thanks for willingness to try something different. Or for the friend who's walking beside you.

Just one or two minutes of silent mental appreciation can change the way you end a walk. Instead of winding down with complaints about how out of shape you are, the walk closes on an up note, a moment of remembering what is still working in your life.

Time to Walk!

OK, put on your walking shoes! Let these guidelines set your course this week. No matter where you begin, you may want to make changes even before the week is over. Extend your walk by a minute or two if you feel more energetic than you expected. Cut back if you feel worn out. Keep in mind that small steps are safe steps. Be kind to yourself by targeting a goal you can achieve.

- Start gently. Begin with a time and a distance that fit into your routine most days of the week.
- If medical advisors have given you guidelines for activity, be responsible in honoring those recommendations.
- If there is any question about your readiness for walking, check with your health team before launching a new program.

- If at any time you find that walking creates increased pain or discomfort, cut back on the distance you walk.
- If physical discomfort persists, this is something to discuss with your medical team; you may need to explore another form of movement, such as swimming or biking.

If you choose to follow the Mid-Stride walking goals this week and find that you are low on energy one day, or tight on time, shorten your walk that day. The Strong and Steady schedule represents an ambitious goal. It is a good pursuit if you are ready for it, but if you find that you are dragging at twenty-five minutes of walking, don't push yourself to do more. If you're accustomed to longer walks on a regular basis, you need not limit walks to times suggested in this program. By adding focusing techniques into your normal walking routine, you'll be enhancing the benefits of your steps, boosting stress release and tranquility.

Take time to write your goals for this week on the Week One log in the appendix of the book, if you haven't already done that. Writing down your intention is like making a contract with yourself. It helps you achieve your goals.

Experiment by rotating the walk outlines at your level during the week to see which approach gets you started most easily. Which focusing technique draws your thoughts away from worries most effectively? Note your responses on the daily log as a way to reinforce your experience.

Week One Goals Overview

Walk Level	Walk Time Goal	Silent Segment Time Goal
Stepping Out	Walk 6 days 10 min. a day	10 min. silent
Mid-Stride	Walk 6 days 20 min. a day	15–20 min. silent
Strong and Steady	Walk 6 days 30 min. a day	20–30 min. silent

A Guided Path to Your Goals

Use these guidelines for walks that meet your goal this week. Rotate the suggested walk outlines to give yourself variety as you practice new focusing techniques. Adjust length of segments to meet your personal time goals. Include a silent segment in every walk.

Week One Daily Walk Guidelines

Stepping Out		
Week 1	Focusing Techniques Rotate routines for variety	Suggested Timing
3 days 10 min.	1. Put Your Foot Down 2. Four-Step: 1-2-3-4 3. Say Thank You	5 min. 3 min. 2 min.
3 days 10 min.	1. Breathe In, Breathe Out 2. Four-Step: 1-2-3-4 3. Say Thank You	3 min. 5 min. 2 min.

Mid-Stride		
Week 1	Focusing Techniques Rotate routines for variety	Suggested Timing
3 days 20 min.	1. Put Your Foot Down 2. Four-Step: 1-2-3-4 3. Say Thank You	8 min. 10 min. 2 min.
3 days 20 min.	1. Breathe In, Breathe Out Or: Walk, Talk, Listen 2. Four-Step: 1-2-3-4 3. Say Thank You	7 min. 10 min. 3 min.

Strong and Steady		
Week 1	Focusing Techniques Rotate routines for variety	Suggested Timing
3 days 30 min.	1. Breathe In, Breathe Out Or: Walk, Talk, Listen 2. Put Your Foot Down 3. Four-Step: 1-2-3-4 4. Say Thank You	8 min. 10 min. 10 min. 2 min.
3 days 30 min.	1. Put Your Foot Down 2. Breathe In, Breathe Out 3. Four-Step: 1-2-3-4 4. Say Thank You	10 min. 5 min. 10 min. 5 min.

Log In

Use the Week One log in the appendix to keep a record of your achievements and discoveries this week. Note your energy level, your walk route, and your experience with this week's focusing techniques.

- How did you feel when you started the walk? Did you feel better, worse, or unchanged at the end?
- Did today's walk impact your mood or energy level? In what way?
- What did you notice when you began to Put Your Foot Down mindfully? Did your posture change when you paid attention to each step?
- Did you find it relaxing to count steps? Boring?
- What did you feel grateful for on this walk?

Of course, you'll miss a day now and then. Medical appointments may stretch longer than planned. You have houseguests from out of town. This happens in life. When you miss a day, you don't have to make it up or feel that you have failed. The real success comes when you walk again the following day. That's a demonstration of your ability to bounce back from a disruption. That's resiliency.

Week Two

A Healthy Spirit

Let the spirit move you this week as you bring increased awareness of breath to your walks. When breath combines with movement and focus, it creates a healing blend that clears the mind and energizes cells. Add the power of cognitive override to support your goals and you'll gain strength that sustains a healing journey.

W as it the artificial sweeteners on my shredded wheat or too many diet sodas? Was it too much estrogen or too few children? Or was it chemicals sprayed on the berries and beans that I picked in my adolescence to earn money for school clothes?

The questions dogged my steps relentlessly on the day I learned that the cancer in my body had spread beyond the tissue of my breast and penetrated lymph nodes as well. My mind ricocheted through factors linked with risk of cancer, seeking a "cause." An explanation. Was it resentment, too long simmering, or small grudges allowed to grow? Was it stress or the festering poison of perfectionism, untempered with compassion? Or the consequences of a type-A personality without the balance of meditation?

The lump was small, I had told myself when a biopsy first confirmed malignancy. Medical opinions were reassuring. Most likely the cancer had not spread. Most likely there would be no need for chemotherapy's full-body assault on mutant cells. Then came medical results that deflated the positive outlook I had clung to through surgery. "You have metastatic cancer." Guilt and blame flooded in to fill the space vacated by optimism. What had I done wrong? What errors led me to this frightening diagnosis? The questions plunged me into a life review in search of something—a decision, a choice, a habit, a person—anything to blame. In search of a place to take control.

I turned, for relief, to a path I knew well. The summit trail in a nearby county park rises steadily through grassy meadows and oak groves for about one and a half miles to the rounded crown of a local hill, a popular route for exercisers, bird lovers, and nature seekers. As I started up the hillside trail, the mental tangle of causes and effects wrapped tight around my mind. *It's not fair!* my brain protested. *There's no cancer in my family. I eat a low-fat diet. I exercise regularly. What did I do to deserve this?*

Everyone who experiences the blow of a difficult diagnosis or a personal crisis encounters an internal interrogation. *Why me? Could I have prevented this? What did I do wrong?* We wrestle with guilt as well as with fear, creating a turmoil of anxiety. We grieve not only the trauma we've encountered, but also the loss of control. Hard times stun us and leave us feeling helpless. Walking offered one small way for me to take action.

On the trail, I wanted to walk away from the questions that pursued me. To quell the mental barrage, I called on a backpacking mantra that had carried me through wilderness camping trips and up yet another switchback when my pack began to feel impossibly heavy. I hoped it would do the same for the load I now carried. *One-step-for-ward-at-a-time,* I chanted mentally as I plodded up the hill. One step per syllable. Each footstep punctuating the phrase. Simple, but so difficult to do. Questions pushed through the tiny pause between one step and the next. *One-step-for-What did I do wrong? One-step-for-ward-What will I do now? One-step-for-Mastectomy?*

Lumpectomy? How to choose? For thirty minutes I fought my way up the trail, returning over and over to the rhythmic mantra that pulled my focus to something I could still control—one step, one breath, and then one more.

By the time I reached the summit, I was breathing hard. I paused to catch my breath and gaze out on the valley below. The farmlands, the freeway, the fork of the river—the view was familiar and reassuring. I'd seen it many times. But on this day, I saw something different. As I looked at the river, I saw a metaphor: When a river gets polluted, we don't ask what the river did to cause it. We don't wonder what the river did to deserve it. We ask what we should do to clean it up!

All the way down the hill I focused on the river. If I could view my body as a waterway, polluted by something outside my control, then I could clean it up and move on. Clean it up and try, as best I could, to avoid further pollution, of course, but first clean it up. The image prepared me to accept chemotherapy as part of the cleansing necessary for this river of my being to live healthy and whole. The metaphor shifted my focus from cause to cure, from helplessness to action. It gave me a grasp of something I could do, one step at a time. It felt like a miracle.

Air + Movement + Focus = Miracle

A thirty-minute walk in nature didn't change the reality of my situation or the seriousness of my disease. It didn't eliminate my fears. But it did settle the chaos in my mind enough that I could see a path through the new landscape before me. It opened my senses and my cells so that I could look into a river and see an image of healing that carried me through nine months of treatment. It enabled me to move forward on a path of cleansing rather than blaming. *That* was a miracle!

In truth, the miracle is breath. The boost in oxygen and circulation that accompanies brisk walking does miraculous things for the human brain. It increases clarity, problem-solving skills, and memory, for starters. But oxygen alone might not have given me the metaphor of a river that enabled me to move forward on a path of cleansing rather than blaming. When I began to chant *one-step-for-ward-at-a-time* in my mind on that hike, I was making a conscious choice to block out a crazy-making swirl of questions, fears, and resentments. That was cognitive override—a crucial ingredient in the mix of movement and air that can lead to a fresh point of view. Each time I returned to the phrase, I was exercising cognitive override to make a willful choice to improve my thinking skills by giving my mind a respite from the battering assault of fear. With a mental chant, I seized control of what I could at a time when so much seemed beyond my grasp.

Cognitive override means using your mental skills to make a choice that is, ultimately, in your best interest.

You're practicing cognitive override on the walks you take in this program. Putting focus on *In* and *Out* as you breathe is a very simple way to take your focus away from mental chatter. This week, you'll expand breath awareness with variations that make each breath a healing cycle of receiving and releasing. The tools are easy, but most people discover that worries soon push to the front again. Some fascinating, important thought will creep around the edges of your mind, even while you are mentally repeating *In* or *Out,* and your thoughts go swirling after it. You're caught in the web again. That's when you need cognitive override. As soon as you notice your mind has moved away from focus on your breath or your steps, you have a choice: to return to a mindful focus or to follow the train of thought that is tempting you. If your intention is to clear your head, or to restore energy and release stress so that your body can focus on healing, you must choose to override the distracting voice. It's a choice you'll make over and over, even on a ten-minute walk. Each time you override a distraction, you are making a choice to take control of one small behavior—a choice that supports your healing.

Robert Thayer, a research psychologist at California State University, Long Beach, developed the concept of cognitive override after studying what makes some people stick with exercise programs while others drop out. The bottom line in predicting lasting success with any exercise program, he says, often turns out to be cognitive override.

"Cognitive override is a term I made up to describe how people can use information from previous experiences to enable them to override a bodily impulse not to engage in activity," Thayer says.[1] "If you are too tired to move, but you know, because you have done it before, that once you start to walk you won't feel as tired, then you can override the impulse to sit. You go exercise even when you don't initially feel like it," he says.

Cognitive override—the use of memory, information, and personal experience—is a process of talking yourself into doing something you know will produce a positive outcome, even though it seems daunting. "Think of cognitive override as muscle strengthening," Thayer says. "There's a learning curve. When you practice something over and over, you learn to do it better."

Cognitive override is perhaps the most valuable tool that you can take from this book. Appreciate it. Remember it. Use it. Cognitive override is not easy or automatic. It always requires a conscious choice to "override" some behavior that seems tempting at the moment—the urge to sleep a few more moments, or check your e-mail instead of going out for a walk. Cognitive override enables you to use your own mental skills to make the choice that is, ultimately, in your own best interest. If you have a job and you need to keep it, it's in your best interest to get up when the alarm goes off, even though you'd love to sleep in. If awareness of calories and sugar intake is important to your health, a second piece of cake is not in your best interest . . . no matter how tempting it sounds at the moment.

If you long for peace of mind, renewed energy, and healthy balance in your life, it's in your best interest to make time for activities, such as walking, that restore wholeness of body, mind, and spirit. When you combine cognitive override with focused breathing and rhythmic movement, you choose a path that makes miracles possible. You clear your mind to see fresh views, as I did when I hiked to a new point of view about my cancer treatment by taking *one-step-for-ward-at-a-time.*

An Air of Determination

Stephen Gaudet knows more than most of us about the significant bond between cognitive override, fresh air, and survival. Born with severe asthma, Stephen grew up wheezing. Hospitalizations punctuated his childhood and isolated him in a social corner where he felt excluded from normal activities and school connections.

"I was embarrassed by my illness," he says.[2] "I had a really bad childhood. I couldn't do anything physical and I hated PE. Having a chronic disease really messes up your self-image." Asthma guided him into a career as a respiratory therapist in San Francisco. As he coached patients to breathe easier, his own disease progressed to "fixed" asthma, a term that indicates permanent, irreparable lung damage, similar to emphysema. His lung capacity hovers at about 36 percent of normal.

At age forty-nine, frequent asthma flare-ups turned Stephen into a patient more often than a therapist. When disability forced him to give up his job, he slumped into weight gain and depression. It took a year of grieving and lethargy before he found the energy to prod himself out of the chair by the television. "Rather than become a couch potato and feeling sorry for myself, I wanted to see if I could slow the progress of my disease with a self-directed fitness regimen, and maybe lose some of the weight I'd gained from steroid treatments," he says.

Using his training as a respiratory therapist and his determination to survive, he set up a personal fitness program. "Exercise is very counterintuitive when you have lung disease, because you can't breathe. But I knew I had to do something," he says. "I had to condition myself to get used to the feeling of being short of breath." He tried biking and jogging but found that both activities left him breathless in a matter of minutes. Walking seemed to be all that he had left, so he started out with a few blocks a day.

He set a daily goal of one-half mile, the round-trip distance from his home on the north shore of San Francisco Bay to the nearest grocery store. Almost anything could make him gasp, even a change in the weather. He carried an inhaler the way that other walkers tote water bottles. Gradually, he pushed his distances until he was walking five miles at a time. And he was beginning to feel good. Beginning to feel like he could do things that normal people do. "I feel like I'm taking an active role in my own health. That makes me feel good about myself."

In 2009, five years after he started walking, Stephen pushed himself beyond "normal" when he became the first severe asthmatic in history to complete the Boston Marathon. His achievement wasn't a race for time as much as a race for respect. To finish the 26.2-mile course, he walked for seven hours and thirty-two minutes, an average pace of 17:22 minutes per mile. It's a snail's pace for marathoners—but a victorious pace for a survivor competing against medical expectations and physical limits.

The achievement did not come without risk. Stephen spent five days in a Boston hospital following the marathon, but does not hesitate when asked if the rewards outweigh the risks in such events. "Absolutely," he says. "How many people with end-stage lung disease have finished the Boston Marathon?"

Some specialists warn that he is living dangerously by tackling marathons, but Stephen credits walking with keeping him alive. "I am absolutely convinced that I would be dead without an exercise program," he says. Medical approval from Stephen's pulmonary specialist was a requirement for participation in the Boston Marathon. The six-hour time limit applied to most participants was waived, making completion, not speed, the record that mattered.

"Walking has opened a new world to me," says Stephen, who entered his first marathon in 2006 and completed three more before gaining entry to the Boston event. "Walking has given me the confidence to do things. Walking definitely made me feel better about myself."

Although walking has not expanded his lung capacity, Stephen's breathing has stabilized, rather than decreased, in recent years. And walking has produced huge increases in other areas of his life. It has opened him to aspirations and fulfillment that carry him beyond the daily rituals that maintain his lungs.

"Everything in my life revolves around my lungs, but there are brief moments when I'm walking that everything clicks and I forget about my lungs and my limitations. I feel like I'm on top of the world. I feel like I'm flying. If I can get that feeling, it's a very good day. I can tell you this, I don't plan on stopping anytime soon."

Taking a Stand for Air

Breathing is something most of us can take for granted. Yes, a long flight of stairs may produce a bit of huffing and puffing. A dash for the bus or a walk up the hills of San Francisco might leave you feeling winded. But unlike Stephen, most of us pay little day-to-day attention to the process that keeps us alive. Breath is the spirit of life. It is both the fuel that sustains our physical existence and the symbol of a spiritual essence larger than our human selves.

Many spiritual traditions acknowledge the significance of breath. Words for breath often have relationship to words that mean spirit. In Latin, the word *spiritus* means both "breath" and "spirit." In Sanskrit, the term *prana* refers to the life force carried in the breath. In English, the words *spirit, inspire, aspire,* and *expire* all share the same core, *spir.* So when we speak of *respiration,* perhaps we are really saying that we are "re-spiriting" ourselves. When we are *inspired,* we feel the spirit move into us. And when someone *expires,* the spirit exits the body. *Aspirations* are goals the spirit moves toward.

If you define breath as life and spirit, wouldn't you aspire to get as much as possible? To *re-spirit* your cells and your soul with full, deep respiration? Yoga, tai chi, relaxation, and meditation all honor the power of breath to enhance physical, mental, and spiritual well-being. The Walking Well program creates a similar merger of body, mind, and spirit. You make the most of this merger of movement and breath when your posture supports full, regular breathing.

As you walk this week, check your posture from time to time. (See page 23 for posture tips.) If you feel short of breath or tired, consider your stature. Have your head and shoulders rolled forward? Is your spine slumped and rounded? If so, you are cutting off breathing space. As you practice the focusing tools this week, you will be increasing the fullness of your breath. Perhaps it will feel unfamiliar to you. In times of fear or stress, breathing patterns become shallow. We hold our breath literally, waiting to see what's coming next. This week, open your mind, and your posture, to fresh air—the catalyst for miracles and mental breakthroughs.

SIDE STEPS: *Walking and Energy*

Too tired to walk? Too down in the dumps to get up on your feet? It happens to all of us. We turn to the refrigerator for a snack and abandon exercise plans. Unfortunately, we let fatigue lead us astray—that snack is not as effective as a walk when it comes to boosting energy and mood.

Just five minutes of walking can reset energy levels, says research psychologist Robert Thayer.[3] In studies at California State University, Thayer found that ten minutes of brisk walking produced more energy than a candy bar, and without the slump that can follow a sugar high. Energy levels remained elevated for up to two hours after a brisk ten-minute walk. Even five minutes of walking has a significant effect on energy.

"It's been shown in many studies that once you actually start moving around—even just getting up off the couch and walking around the room—the more you will want to move, and the more energy you will feel," says Thayer. "Even five minutes. You will feel it."

For the biggest boost in the shortest time, Thayer recommends a walking pace that forces you to hurry a little. Imagine you are headed for an appointment and don't want to be late. You have time to reach your destination, but you can't be lazy about it.

The benefits of that brisk walk become even more convincing when you consider the significant correlation between energy and mood. Energy is a core component of mood. When energy is up, moods tend to lift. When energy drops, so does temperament. What's more, energy is an indicator of mental and physical well-being.[4]

Unfortunately, it's hard to do the very thing that can help the most when your energy is low. But knowledge is power. When you know in your head, and through experience, that walking leads to improved energy and emotional state, you are better prepared to override the downward pull of a hard time.

Sedentary people who engage in a regular exercise program consistently experience improved energy and reduced fatigue, according to researchers at the University of Georgia who analyzed seventy studies involving more than 6,800 people.[5] The results were consistent across a broad range of participants, including healthy adults, cancer patients, heart disease patients, people with mental health problems, and persons battling recurring fatigue.

Although the impetus to get up and move starts in your head, the energy that exercise produces isn't all in your mind. It comes from chemical reactions in cells throughout the body. When circulation is stimulated by movement, oxygen rushes through the body, triggering energy production by tiny organs called mitochondria, located within the cells. The more you exercise, the more mitochondria the body produces. Regular exercise is a way to train the cells to retain a higher number of mitochondria, thus boosting your supply of energy. When you wonder if a walk is worth the effort, remind yourself that your body is producing mitochondria—little energy engines—as you walk. Think about the biological chemistry that allows you to build a more robust source of internal power just by taking this walk.

To keep a lamp burning, we have to keep putting oil in it.

—Mother Teresa

We all know it takes fuel to keep just about everything in working condition. That fuel might be oil, as in the lamp that Mother Teresa mentions in her remark, above. It might be the gas to keep the car moving. Or the fuel we take in as food—the nourishment that gives us strength and energy to function day by day.

But our bodies need another kind of fuel as well. Air is the fuel of life. Without it, we won't last long. Because breath is always with us, it is a common focusing tool for meditation. Steady, deep breathing calms the mind and relaxes muscles. But athletes also learn to focus on breath. This week's walks will expand on the techniques that you practiced last week by adding breathing patterns that enhance stress release while fueling your cells.

How you breathe is not as important as *that* you breathe. The goal is to fill your lungs with air, gently expanding your body's capacity for life. If it is comfortable to breathe through your nose, inhale and exhale through the nose. That is the purpose of the nose, after all. I find that I breathe in and out through my nose when I am walking at a moderate pace. When I speed up to raise my heart rate, I tend to breathe in through the nose and out through my mouth. Feel free to experiment. There is no right or wrong, so long as you get a full breath.

This week's walks give you a variety of breathing and focusing techniques. Try them all. Some exercises may seem uncomfortable. You may find that you need to adjust the rate or depth of your respiration. Experiment. Push your judgment aside and give each exercise a chance. Only by experimenting can you discover new tools that will assist you in restoring balance and movement in your life.

Remember that silence is a valuable component of healing. In silence you allow yourself to reconnect with your own values, priorities, and needs. You begin to restore wholeness by healing the splits that separate your "being" and your "doing." Probably you've said it yourself. If not, you've surely thought it: *I'm so rattled I can't even hear myself think. What I need is a little peace and quiet!* Yet we do almost everything we can to avoid silence. We have become accustomed to surrounding ourselves with noise at all times. Learning to be comfortable with silence is sometimes challenging. But if you seek healing that is more than physical, make a choice to honor silence in walks that become a moving meditation.

When you walk with a partner, use the optional Walk, Talk, Listen segments included in longer walks below. Then practice walking together in silent support as you turn your attention to mental focusing techniques that help clear your path.

1. FOUR-STEP: IN-2-3-4 CADENCE

Last week, you practiced counting footsteps as a way to keep mind and body together on your walks. This week, you are going to add another dimension to the count by creating a four-count cadence that links words, steps, and breath. Begin as you did last week, counting your steps in a pattern of one-two-three-four. When you have the rhythm, modify the words slightly so you are mentally saying *In-two-three-four, Out-two-three-four.* Match your breathing with the words. Inhale for four steps and exhale for four steps. The inhalation is equal to the exhalation. Maybe you did that last week, automatically. Sometimes it happens without awareness. But this week, be conscious of the rhythm that unites breath, steps, and mental focus.

Most people are not accustomed to a regular, balanced pattern of breathing—taking in as much air as you let out, and releasing as much as you took in. It may feel unusual at first, but it's an important metaphor for the way we live. If you don't practice taking in as much fuel as you expend, at least some of the time, how can you sustain your own vitality? If you don't let out the stale air that is locked inside, how can you make room for fresh air or fresh inspiration?

2. CLEAR THE AIR

Clear your head when you set out on a walk by using your breath as a vehicle for releasing stress and bringing in new, vibrant energy. As you inhale, imagine that you are drawing in new life, new awareness, new opportunities, new courage to move forward in life. As you exhale, imagine that all the stale, used-up residue in your cells is flowing out of you. Exhale slowly. Whatever you want to release, feel it loosening and letting go with your breath.

This exercise is a wonderful way to let go of problems that follow you out on your walks. Use it to get present in the moment, breathing in new life and releasing what you no longer need or want to hold on to. If you notice that your mind wanders off to pursue something old as you are releasing it, you may find it helpful to insert a four-step cadence that helps your mind stay focused. Try saying to yourself, *Fresh air comes in. Stale air goes out.* The phrases maintain the four-count pattern—four syllables, four steps. But now you have a new focus. See if you can actually feel fresh energy coming into your body as your mind states *Fresh air comes in.* Can you feel the circulation of air into your lungs and imagine it moving through your muscles? When you exhale, saying *Stale air goes out,* feel your body relax and release tension, anger, weariness. You are also releasing carbon dioxide—a by-product no longer useful to your cells. It is a strong image as you are stepping forward, opening to life.

When you lose focus and find your mind racing away, remind yourself, *Not now.* Return your focus to breathing. *Not now* is cognitive override. It gives you the power to overrule the impulsive part of your brain that is easily distracted.

3. YIN-YANG BREATH: EARTH AND SKY

In the traditional Chinese approach to qi gong, movement is regarded as a component of healing. "Qi" (or chi) represents breath, spirit, or core energy that sustains life. "Qi gong" is the art of managing one's breathing to achieve and maintain good health. This exercise brings a qi gong variation to the previous practice of drawing in fresh energy and releasing stale air. Qi gong teaches that the earth, the surface that supports us as we walk, holds yin energy—the energy of receptivity. The sky holds yang energy—the energy of action. We need both kinds of energy to be healthy and balanced living beings.

For this exercise, imagine that you are inhaling a spirit of receptivity. Receptivity does not mean passivity. I imagine receptivity as openness, willingness to explore new concepts or thoughts, courage to listen to myself and to the wisdom that guides me. Perhaps you want to be receptive to love, or to creativity, or trust. Let it flow into you, rising up from the earth through your feet and legs as you inhale.

As you exhale, imagine that the energy of action—brain energy, problem solving, forward movement—is pouring into the top of your head from the sky. Feel it flow down your neck and shoulders and arms. Imagine that it carries the strength to take the next step. The clarity to make the next decision. Let it flow through your cells. Then inhale again, drawing in earth energy—openness and receptivity.

How does your body feel as you do this exercise? Can you sense how you need both giving and receiving? Doing and being? So often, a traumatic event or illness severs that give and take. We can get caught in the "fight or flight" response that triggers more stress. This exercise helps restore a balanced, cooperative relationship of mind, body, and spirit.

Previous Exercises You'll Use This Week

As you acquire additional focusing techniques, the mindfulness options available for you on walks will be expanding. This week, your walks include exercises from last week. Look back at descriptions in the Walking Well section of Week One if you want to refresh your memory. It may be helpful to jot down an outline of the walk to carry with you.

1. BREATHE IN, BREATHE OUT (WEEK ONE)

Continue practicing this exercise from last week. Mentally say *In* as you inhale a full, deep breath of air. As you exhale, say *Out*. The mental prompts of *In, Out* help you stay focused on each breath.

2. PUT YOUR FOOT DOWN (WEEK ONE)

Make smooth contact with the surface that supports you by using each foot as a rocker. Smooth out your steps by touching down with your heel first and rolling forward to the toes. Notice your full foot, feeling the solid connection with the surface that holds you up.

3. SAY THANK YOU (WEEK ONE)

Conclude each walk with a few moments of appreciation. Acknowledge your own willingness to experiment and take the risk to open your lungs, and your imagination.

Week Two Goals Overview

Walk Level	Walk Time Goal	Silent Segment Time Goal
Stepping Out	Walk 6 days 10–12 min. a day	10 min. silent
Mid-Stride	Walk 6 days 20 min. 4–5 days 25 min. 1–2 days	15–20 min. silent
Strong and Steady	Walk 6 days 30 min. 5–6 days Optional: 40 min. 1 day	20–30 min. silent

Week Two Daily Walk Guidelines

As you start the second week of your walking program, renew your agreement with yourself by choosing goals you can achieve. You want to feel successful in making movement a regular part of your daily life. Write your goals on the Week Two log in the appendix. If you discovered that you could easily walk the distances you chose last week, try adding a minute or two this week. Adjust the suggested times as desired to meet your personal goals.

As you walk, you are creating healthy habits and learning skills of resiliency. But learning requires patience and practice. No matter what technique you use, the goal is always to bring mind and body together, working in unison. That is what helps release tension and stress. That is what gets you back on both feet when life slips out of balance.

Stepping Out		
Week 2	Focusing Techniques Rotate routines for variety	Suggested Timing
2 days 10–12 min.	1. Breathe In, Breathe Out 2. Four-Step: In-2-3-4 Cadence 3. Say Thank You	5 min. 5 min. 2 min.
2 days 10–12 min.	1. Clear the Air 2. Four-Step: In-2-3-4 Cadence 3. Say Thank You	5 min. 5 min. 2 min.
2 days 10–12 min.	1. Put Your Foot Down 2. Yin-Yang Breath: Earth and Sky 3. Say Thank You	5 min. 5 min. 2 min.

Mid-Stride		
Week 2	Focusing Techniques Rotate routines for variety	Suggested Timing
4–5 days 20 min.	1. Breathe In, Breathe Out Or: Optional Walk, Talk, Listen 2. Four-Step: In-2-3-4 Cadence 3. Put Your Foot Down 4. Say Thank You	7 min. 5 min. 5 min. 3 min.

(continued on the next page)

Mid-Stride		
Week 2	**Focusing Techniques** Rotate routines for variety	**Suggested Timing**
1–2 days 25 min.	1. Clear the Air Or: Optional Walk, Talk, Listen 2. Four-Step: In-2-3-4 Cadence 3. Yin-Yang Breath: Earth and Sky 4. Say Thank You	10 min. 5 min. 5 min. 5 min.

Strong and Steady		
Week 2	**Focusing Techniques** Rotate routines for variety	**Suggested Timing**
5–6 days 30 min.	1. Breathe In, Breathe Out Or: Optional Walk, Talk, Listen 2. Four-Step: In-2-3-4 Cadence 3. Yin-Yang Breath: Earth and Sky 4. Say Thank You	10 min. 10 min. 5 min. 5 min.
Optional 40 min.	1. Clear the Air Or: Optional Walk, Talk, Listen 2. Put Your Foot Down 3. Four-Step: In-2-3-4 Cadence 4. Yin-Yang Breath: Earth and Sky 5. Say Thank You	10 min. 5 min. 10 min. 10 min. 5 min.

Log In

Remember to record your walks in the Week Two log. The record is like a pat on the back, acknowledging your success in getting your feet back on the ground. Make notes of what you noticed and how you felt, as well as how many times you walked.

- Did you find one exercise especially helpful? Why?
- Did you breathe comfortably with the four-count cadence for steps and breath?

- Could you imagine releasing stale energy from your cells and inhaling fresh air and fresh life? What about yin and yang energy?
- How was your energy level at the beginning and end of the walk?
- What do you give thanks for today?

Week Three

A Healthy Mind

Be mindful of self-talk this week as you pair your steps with words that combat stress and renew spirit. Experience the power of language to support your goals and release doubts. By changing inner dialogue, you lighten your steps, physically, mentally, and spiritually. If you can talk yourself out of a walk, you can also talk yourself into one!

Without the dog, Terry Gray might not have walked the healing path on the hill above the cemetery. Without the dog, he might not have felt the solid footing of the old wagon trail down to the church. Without the dog, he might have withdrawn from the world, might have wrapped himself in grief and rage at the death of his son, Kit.

Josie wouldn't let that happen. Josie was Kit's dog—a Black Mouth Cur found sick and abandoned at a service station. Kit gathered the hunting dog pup up in his arms and carried her home to join other strays he couldn't turn his back on. But Kit couldn't rescue himself. At age twenty-nine, he lost a seventeen-year struggle with drug abuse and died of a heroin overdose. He left behind a bereft family and a pair of forsaken dogs.

"About the second day after his death, it hit me that the dogs had to be walked," says his father.[1] Josie and Domino had worked their way indoors as house dogs, making regular walks an obvious necessity. Domino, a ten-year-old Canaan dog with a big personality and an easy manner, let the younger Josie initiate the walks. Three or four times a day Josie prodded Terry from the numbness of his grief and guided him down the rural road beyond their East Tennessee home. Sometimes she led him up the hill to the cemetery. Sometimes she took him into the ten-acre hollow that lay beyond the house. Past the graveled parking lot where the trucks of Kit's tree-pruning business sat idle.

"Within the first week, it hit me that this was good for me," says Terry. "I've seen people with depression get totally immobilized and unable to get out of bed. I didn't want that, and this was at least getting me moving. I held on to that thought—It's getting me moving, getting me moving."

Soon the walks established a pattern. The dogs took Terry out for strolls that didn't last long—less than a mile most of the time. But they imposed a structure on days that had lost reason and routine. "I suppose I was depressed," he says. "I had trouble focusing on a lot of things."

In some ways, Kit's death was not unexpected. His battle with drugs and emotional turmoil had been a chronic challenge. At age twelve, he entered drug rehabilitation treatment for the first time. It took ten years and two more drug programs before he seemed to gain control of his life. He completed his GED and bought a tree-care business. To support their son's new hold on life, Terry and Karen Gray moved to a farm with acreage that offered space for Kit's work vehicles. A home-based antique business allowed them to spend more time with Kit. But the needles that had pumped Kit's young body with drugs and tattoos transmitted a second hazard. By the time he was diagnosed with hepatitis C, the disease had damaged his liver. He needed an organ transplant.

"He was in a lot of pain," says Terry. "He didn't want to go through a transplant. We were waiting for something to happen, but I wasn't expecting a return to drugs. I don't know when he decided he needed heroin again."

The overdose—by accident or choice is uncertain—stripped Terry and Karen of priorities that had defined their lives for years. Kit's dogs moved forward to offer a new role, and Terry picked up the leash.

"For a whole year I was doing these walks for the dogs' exercise, and for a chance to be alone with my thoughts," he says. "I thought and thought and thought. My brain was working overtime. I thought about the war on drugs and about the judicial system. I thought about everything under the sun."

Then, after a year or so of replaying the same thoughts, the same disappointments, the same anger, Terry tired of prowling the mental maze. He decided to pay attention to the environment and the world around him, rather than focus on the raging commentaries in his head. Domino had wearied of the outings, leaving Josie to guide Terry's walks. As he followed the dog, Terry watched her body language and focused on the same things she did. When she heard a sound, he listened, too. When she stopped and observed, he did the same.

"It got me out of my head for a while. I would just sort of take her perspective on the walk and it seemed a lot more interesting. I would have thought I would get tired of it, but I didn't. My health improved and I started almost depending on these walks."

"After four years of healing through walking, I have come to realize that walking is my practice, and my peace."

By choosing to approach each walk in the way that Josie did, Terry gave his mind a new focus. Observation broke his cycle of fixation on problems by shifting awareness to the present. It's a formula for healing that has been handed down for centuries. The Buddha is reported to have advised listeners that "the secret of health for both mind and body is not to mourn for the past, not to worry about the future, not to anticipate troubles, but to live in the present moment wisely and earnestly."

Terry had read such words before. As a student, he'd delved into philosophy and spiritual values in pursuit of a graduate degree in pastoral counseling. But it took a jarring tragedy and a patient dog to lift the lessons off the page. "For years, I had been looking for guidance in books," he says. "I had been analyzing everything. Josie got me out of that. What she taught me, we have heard for a thousand years: Your teacher is inside yourself.

"After four years of healing through walking, I have come to realize that walking is my practice, my discipline, and my peace," he says. "The walks have taught me trust. Trusting life. Trusting my body. I have received a gift that will last me a lifetime, and that has returned joy into my life."

A Fine Balance

The first words that flared in Terry Gray's head at the tragic death of his son were words of outrage and helplessness. Mentally, he raged against a "war on drugs" that had failed his family completely. He haggled over ways to combat a system that had let his son down. His rage is understandable, perhaps even appropriate. Anger can fuel acts of courage and confrontation with injustice.

Martin Seligman, a psychology professor at the University of Pennsylvania, maintains that there is nothing wrong with negative emotions. Negative words and emotions such as fear, sadness, or anger warn us that something is not right, he says. They mobilize us to take action, stimulating the classic "fight or flight" response. In his book *Authentic Happiness*, Seligman calls that a "battle station" mode of thinking in which all attention goes into identifying what is wrong and getting rid of it. It is an appropriate reaction to many of life's challenges, especially in situations that call for analytical problem solving. A negative mood jolts us into one type of thinking about a situation. A positive mood produces an entirely different approach. Positive moods and thought patterns encourage us to look for what is right. They lead us to explore possibilities and seek creative solutions to situations. In a balanced, successful life, we benefit from both types of thinking. Because negative and positive thoughts activate different areas of the brain, we maximize coping skills and personal happiness by using both. We are more resourceful and more resilient. The "negative" process of analytical, problem-solving thinking provides clarity in an emergency; the "positive" perspective contributes creative thinking, expansive possibilities, and tolerance.[2]

Often, well-meaning friends and family push us to "look on the bright side" of things. They urge us to maintain a positive attitude and warn that negative thinking will bring further illness and pain. While it is true that positive thinking is a valuable tool, it is also true that human beings hold a broad range of emotions, and even negative feelings can have positive value. Being stuck in either "it's all bad" or "everything's rosy" is equally limiting. Balance does not eliminate clear, cold, analytical thinking. It recognizes and utilizes the contribution of both analysis and openness. The key to resiliency and resourcefulness in a crisis is being able to use our full range of mental abilities.

When Terry could acknowledge personal benefits emerging from his walks, he began to restore emotional balance. Simply by telling himself, *It's getting me moving, getting me moving,* he shifted focus away from rage for a few minutes, and toward recovery. The words formed an affirmation that helped him inch forward with an emerging sense of purpose. Steps and words together shaped a path of cautious advance, back into a life that is balanced enough to hold peace and joy as well as grief and loss.

Your walks this week will focus on confronting self-talk patterns that limit your own thinking and healing. As you become aware of the words that circle unbidden through your head, you create opportunities to balance painful patterns with words of support or comfort. When patterns have become entrenched, through years of repetition or the dark burden of depression, it takes commitment to healing, and an act of willpower, to invite the positive back into your life.

Dogged Determination

"Take a walk," social worker Jacqueline Meehan advises depression sufferers who come to her office for counseling. She speaks from personal experience. Depression began to muffle her own vitality while she was in her teens and still lingers in the shadows of her life. When she listens to clients describing the fatigue and numbness of depression, the struggle resonates. In spite of research that solidly confirms the power of walking to lessen symptoms of depression, even a mental health professional can face days when the hurdles seem insurmountable.

"Sometimes I still have days when I just sit on the couch and say, 'I don't feel like it,'" Jacqueline concedes.[3] "Usually I can talk myself into taking a walk, but when you are really depressed, it's true, it's hard to get up and do something for yourself."

On days like that, she counts on cognitive override, previous experience, and on Cinnamon, her cockapoo, to provide the extra tug of motivation that gets her up and moving. As she walks the dog, she recites positive affirmations, choosing a word or phrase that calms a current fear. Sometimes she imagines that she is inhaling life and exhaling pain.

"When the walk ends, I already feel better. I usually have more energy after the walk. I feel more positive," she says.

Jacqueline had learned to regulate her depression with medication and exercise when cervical cancer hurled her back into despair. At age thirty-six, she underwent treatment that freed her of cancer but stripped her of the opportunity to bear a child. She was deep into the grief and depression of a changed life vision when she participated in a walking workshop at a Tucson cancer resource center. The workshop introduced focusing skills that draw attention to breath or positive self-talk and away from fear or grief.

I am healthy, I am strong, she began to repeat mentally as she walked with the workshop group. The words shaped a positive self-image that stilled self-doubt and forged an enduring mantra that Jacqueline relies on when depression darkens her trust in life. "I have always liked walking, but now my walks have more focus," she says, five years after the workshop. "I love using affirmations when I walk. They change my thinking, which changes my emotions. I feel more connected; it's more like prayer."

At age forty-one, Jacqueline considers cancer behind her, but clinical depression remains a chronic, chemical condition.

Walking holds a core position in an ongoing health regimen that includes yoga, acupuncture, and medication. "One way to manage depression is with medicine, and one is with exercise. I don't think medicine alone is a solution," she says. "I feel healthier mentally, emotionally, and physically when I walk. I feel more centered and have more self-esteem, like I am doing something good for myself. I am more focused."

Jacqueline's success in managing depression rests on a two-pronged approach to healing. Consistent exercise is as important as consistent medication in supporting her well-being. The affirmations that ground her provide a life buoy that keeps her afloat when waves of despair roll over her. *I am healthy, I am strong.* She grasps the words firmly in hard times, and sidesteps a mental search for reasons or answers or blame. *I am healthy, I am strong.* In taking control of the thoughts in her head, even for a few moments, she creates an opening for healing.

A Word to the Wise

Cardiologist Herbert Benson, MD, is a pioneering researcher in mind-body healing and in the impact of stress on the human body. Much of his work has investigated the effectiveness of exercise and meditation or prayer in releasing stress and reducing the risks that accumulate when stress becomes a way of life. Although we blame the pressures of modern life for filling our lives with stress, Benson cautions that the greatest threat is actually from forces inside. Much of the stress people feel, he says, comes from the way we talk to ourselves. We replay an endless mental loop of badgering criticism and self-judgment:

I'm too old . . . too sick . . . too weak . . . too poor . . . too dumb . . . too fat . . . too busy . . . too short . . . too tired . . . etc.

Benson has a very dramatic description for this process. He says that most of us "marinate our minds in negativity."[4] I love the powerful, visual image these words create. It's easy to imagine my poor, beleaguered brain soaking in a murky marinade of self-criticism, comparison, dissatisfaction, shoulds, and fears. What's worse, says Benson, I am the one who continues to stir that marinade. I have forgotten that I could simply *change* the marinade any time I wanted. All I have to do is stir up a blend of fresh ingredients—new words, new thoughts, new images.

Richard Davidson, a neuroscientist at the University of Wisconsin–Madison, has done research confirming that positive thoughts stimulate the same area of the brain as meditation practices do. People who practice positive thinking demonstrate benefits in health and stress release similar to those seen in people who meditate. Put Davidson's results together with Herbert Benson's suggestion that negative self-talk is the culprit producing most of the stress in the human body, and it makes sense to give your brain a change of marinade once in a while.

But how to do it? It's not easy to break mental habits, and it's almost never a simple matter of saying, "No self-judgment allowed." In fact, the process of fighting back negative thoughts can be stress-inducing in itself. Even many forms of meditation suggest focusing on the words of a mantra or a prayer rather than struggling to clear the mind completely. Athletes also learn to crowd out thoughts of doubt and judgment with positive images or words. They baste their brains with powerful, positive marinades and support their goals with words of confidence.

When runner Nick Symmonds trained for the qualifying meet that would decide his chance to compete in the 2008 Olympics in Beijing, his anxiety grew daily. "There was a constant battle between the part of me that wondered if I was training too hard, and the part that feared I wasn't training hard enough," he says. "Perhaps the toughest hurdle came when I began to question whether I was really Olympic material." He combated the doubts by turning his thoughts to athletes whose determination and dedication had inspired his athletic goals, and with words that supported his own efforts: "I am now prepared physically and mentally to prove that I belong on the 2008 Olympic team." The affirmation turned out to be true. Nick ran in Beijing as a member of the U.S. Olympic Team. Although he did not bring home a medal in his first Olympic appearance, he achieved a goal of representing his country as one of the world's top athletes.[5]

Silencing Pain

The woman who approached me at the conclusion of a walking workshop in Hot Springs, Virginia, had tears in her eyes. We had just returned from a walk in which I introduced participants to the mental focusing tools you are learning—to walk in silence, to pay attention to breathing in and breathing out, to count steps—tools that help the body release stress and also enable the mind to be more consciously present in the moment, aware of the world around and within.

For many years, she said, she had cherished solitary walks in the countryside near her home. Those walks provided a welcome break in busy days. But after the death of her husband, words of loss and sorrow careened through her mind anytime she took her attention off work and ventured out on a walk alone. In recent years she had rigorously avoided walking by herself. She came to a walkers' rally because it offered opportunities to hike in a group of like-minded people with whom she could visit. Only by talking as she walked was she able to push aside the sadness that poured itself into every silent moment.

She had almost bolted, she admitted, when I asked the group to experiment with walking in silence. She felt the panic tighten her chest. She wanted to turn and walk away. To be polite, she stayed, and in the process she discovered a detour around the voices in her head. *I am here and I am strong. I am here and I am walking,* she chanted mentally as the group walked through autumn woods in silence. *I am here and I am strong. I am here and I am walking,* she repeated, using words of a chant as a buffer against the spiral of grief she had come to expect in any opening.

Each repetition of the phrase demonstrated an act of cognitive override, an act of choice and control. Each repetition represented a conscious choice to banish words of loneliness, helplessness, vulnerability, just for a few minutes at a time. Long enough to let her body restore balance and her cells to rediscover comfort and renewal in silence.

In that one walk, she said, she found a tool that freed her to walk again. She learned to push aside fear at being alone in the world by substituting words of strength and trust. The words, and the silent walk, led her to a turning point. Not forgetting the man who had shared her love and her life, but learning how to move forward on a new path, no longer trapped by pain.

Affirmative Action

This week, exercises in the Walking Well program will help you change habitual mental patterns by creating a new "marinade." The change begins with learning to hear your own negative self-talk and then taking action to stop it. For me, the fastest way to interrupt self-talk has been to insert a new set of words. By counting footsteps mentally, or chanting or reciting a meaning-ful phrase in my mind, I block the intrusion of stressful thoughts and my walk becomes an active, walking meditation that refuels both body and spirit.

Another word for a positive marinade might be affirmation. An affirmation is a phrase you can say or write to counteract negative self-talk. "Yes, I can," is an affirmation that refutes the whiny, internal voice that thinks you are too tired to walk today. It is an affirmation of determination, and of commitment. Maybe you walk slowly. Maybe you walk a shortened route. But when you tell yourself, "Yes, I can," you affirm mental and physical strength to stay on a healing path.

Words are the key ingredient in a new mental marinade. When affirmations, prayer, or mantras become part of your regu-lar walks, the words you repeat slide into your cells, restoring the connection of body, mind, and spirit. The rhythmic repetition of words and movement deepens mental relaxation, allowing brain patterns to merge with body patterns. You begin a journey that is simultaneously internal and external, gently healing the mind-body split that so often accompanies illness or trauma.

Rhythmic repetition of words and movement deepens mental relaxation, gently healing the mind-body split that often occurs with illness or trauma.

Often, affirmations are statements, such as "I am strong" or "I am healthy." They affirm a condition that you seek to expand in your life. We all can say, "I am strong" and feel the energy of the words. It doesn't mean we have impressive bicep muscles, or that we can do physical labor all day. But we may have a strong will to live, a strong desire to feel better, a strong commitment to goals. "I am strong" is a true statement that affirms something we want to honor and perhaps expand.

"I am healthy" may feel like a lie when one has just received a troubling medical diagnosis. But try saying it as an affirmation of a condition you want to amplify in your life and you may begin to notice that parts of you are clearly healthy. Perhaps you have a healthy head of hair. Healthy lungs. A healthy brain. A healthy appetite. By mentally repeating the affirmative phrase "I am healthy," it's possible to confront the tendency to catastrophize. When we put total attention on what has gone wrong, we quickly lose sight of things that are still OK. Of course, it's essential to look at what needs to be healed, but it's also valuable to find time to shift the focus, and the stress, so that you can restore balance.

Daily walks offer an opportunity to practice balance in both body and mind. Some people are skeptical of affirmations and regard positive self-talk as "pie in the sky" fantasies. The solution to that concern is to create realistic affirmations. For instance, I can affirm that "I am tall," even though my height is very average. "Tall" can be a description of my posture and of the way I carry myself when I walk. But I can't affirm that "I am six feet tall" and expect to get positive results. That would be pie in the sky. Likewise, I can't affirm, "I am cured of cancer." I don't know if I am free from cancer cells in my body. I know that I am symptom free. I know that I am healthy by current medical measurements. I can affirm that I am healthy, but not that I am cured.

As you walk this week, experiment with focusing techniques that encourage you to create positive mental statements. Try out words that support and energize you rather than build stress in your body. Choose outcomes that you believe are attainable. If you are more comfortable thinking of mental marinade as prayer, rather than affirmation, that is equally effective. The key is to find words that uplift you while blocking out words of fear or anger. If you find comfort in spiritual scriptures, choose a phrase that is meaningful to you.

The sooner you can shift focus away from negative notions about yourself, the better you'll walk and feel. In a study at Yale University, researchers found that a positive image or feelings of appreciation energized walkers to move faster, increasing the benefits of exercise.[6] Next time you catch yourself thinking *I'm too tired, too slow, too out of shape*, remember that negative self-talk is a heavy weight that robs you of energy.

SIDE STEPS: *Walking and Mood*

When you feel the least like moving—when your mood is desolate and your energy depleted—the medicine that can ease your pain may be hard to swallow. Psychiatrist and Harvard Medical School professor John Ratey calls exercise "the psychiatrist's dream treatment." As little as ten minutes of walking, at a pace brisk enough to raise a sweat, has a beneficial effect, he says.[7]

Significant changes in depression symptoms show up with a few weeks of regular exercise, about the same amount of time it takes antidepressant drugs to work, Ratey says. "And we are talking about seriously ill people here—the clinically depressed. They are responding to exercise."

Depressive disorders affect almost 10 percent of the U.S. population aged eighteen and older, reports the National Institute of Mental Health. Nearly twice as many women as men are affected by depression. Evidence supporting exercise as a treatment for depression and mood disorders is growing as neuroscience explores the chemistry of the brain.

Exercise helps combat depression because it stimulates the

production of neurotransmitters that are known to affect mood—norepinephrine, serotonin, and dopamine. Exercise regulates these chemicals in much the same way as many antidepressant medications, and, often, just as effectively.

MOVEMENT AS MEDICINE

When scientists at Duke University Medical Center tested exercise against the antidepressant medication Zoloft, they found that the two were equally successful in reducing or eliminating symptoms of major depressive disorder.[8] Participants in the four-month study exercised with brisk walking, jogging, or stationary bike riding for forty-five minutes, three times a week. Six months after the initial test period, participants in the exercise group were much less likely to have experienced a return of depression than participants treated with medication.

"For each fifty-minute increment of exercise, there was an accompanying 50 percent reduction in relapse risk," says lead researcher James Blumenthal. "The more one exercised, the less likely one would see their depressive symptoms return."

SHAKE A FUNK

At the University of Wisconsin, psychiatrist John Griest found similar results for people with moderate depression. Participants who walked or jogged three times a week for periods of forty-five to sixty minutes at a time reported longer-lasting relief from depression than people treated with medications. Both groups reported relief of symptoms at the end of the twelve-week supervised study, but one year later, people who had been treated with exercise therapy were twice as likely to remain free of depression.[9]

MOVE A MOOD

Psychologist Robert Thayer calls exercise "the single best way of changing a bad mood."[10] Moods shift because exercise produces an increase in energy and a decrease in tension or stress. If you doubt it, Thayer suggests an experiment the next time you are feeling listless and emotionally low. Rate your energy level on a scale of one to seven, with seven being your maximum, feel-good energy level. Then go for a brisk ten-minute walk. At the end of ten minutes, rate your energy again. Probably you will note an increase. This is important, he says, because energy is a core element of mood, and mood is a key index of physical and psychological well-being.

SIDE STEPS: *Fifteen-Minute Mood Mender*

Sometimes, when the pull of a bad mood begins to obscure your view, or a wave of doubt washes over you, there's a moment of choice. Do you make an effort to push away from the current, or surrender to the tides of melancholy? Resistance is never easy, but when you're armed with information and awareness, you stand a chance of resisting a downward eddy.

Try this fifteen-minute mood-mender walk whenever you feel hopeless or helpless. Substitute it for the walk outlined in your weekly Walking Well schedule anytime you need it. Make it a second walk if you are physically fit for a daily double. The key is ten minutes of up-tempo walking that raises heart and respiration rates slightly. To get the results outlined in the Walking and Moods Side Steps, you need to boost circulation and stimulate the release of peptides—the body's natural, feel-good chemicals.

1. *Three-minute warm-up:* Walk at a steady, easy pace. Focus on breathing by mentally repeating *In-Out* as you inhale and exhale.

2. *Ten-minute speed-up:* Pick up the tempo. This should feel like an effort. Try to sustain a pace you would use when late for an appointment. Pull thoughts away from complaints by mentally counting *In-two-three-four, Out-two-three-four.* A cadence strengthens cooperation of mind, muscles, and breath.

3. *Two-minute warm-down:* Slow to a steady, easy walking pace. Mentally, return to *In-Out* to regulate your breathing as you gently return to a normal respiration rate.

Mood-mender walks offer modest miracles. Maybe the changes are subtle, but the healing of movement and circulation often fuel you for wiser choices at the end of the walk. And the benefits are cumulative. Trust the research and give it a try when the doubter within darkens your day.

Language has the power to alter perception.
We think in words, and these words have
the power to limit us or to set us free.

—Dan Baker, *What Happy People Know*

As you move into the third week of Walking Well, you can probably think back on the last two weeks and recognize the power of language in your life. You've been learning to notice the mental chatter that erupts as you walk. Maybe you are becoming more aware of the incessant babble of self-talk that follows your every step through the day. An active brain is a good thing. But an active brain is like an active body—both perform better if they get some rest.

Imagine spending day and night with someone who constantly worried that something horrible might happen. Or someone who second-guessed and criticized every decision you made. And what about someone who warned of disaster at every turn? Imagine that it just never stopped! No break from all this fear and worry. You'd soon feel worn out, stressed out, and frayed. You probably know the feeling. Traumatic events release an eruption of worry, fear, uncertainty, and gloom.

Terry Gray pushed aside the language of disaster on his walks by chanting words of hope: "At least it's getting me moving, getting me moving." Jacqueline Meehan blocks the words of depression with language she calls prayer: "I am healthy, I am strong."

When you can actively pair your steps with words that stop the buzz of fear or anger, you speed the healing process. It doesn't mean you must "pretend" everything is OK. You don't need to put on a happy face. You simply need to give yourself a time-out from the words and fears that spread stress through your body. Even a moment or two of tranquility allows the cells to stop tensing for attack and begin the work of recovery.

This week, you'll add self-talk tools to the mindfulness techniques from the first two weeks of walks. Along with breath and cadence, you'll experiment with words that enable you to "change the marinade" that steeps your brain in anxiety.

The following mindfulness skills are new this week and build on tools you've already learned. Read through the description of each activity and then put words to work for you in your daily walks. Check your posture as you start every walk. Are you standing up straight? Shoulders relaxed and arms swinging freely at your sides? And remember to breathe! Good posture opens the lungs and passageways to receive fresh air, which sets off an energizing chemical change in your cells.

1. THREE-STEP: IN-2-3 CADENCE

This exercise is a lively and invigorating variation on the four-beat cadence walking you have already done. The four-count is a familiar march rhythm, which makes it a great starting point for coordinating steps, breath, and feet. The three-count demands a bit more focus because it is an odd number. You definitely have to stay focused as you shift to breathing in for three counts, and then breathing out for three counts. Mentally, repeat to yourself, *In-two-three, Out-two-three* so you set the rhythm in your mind as well as with your feet.

This may feel awkward at first. That's not surprising when you are learning something new. Be patient. If you feel as if you are breathing too fast, slow it down. Regulate the amount of air you inhale and exhale so that it's comfortable within the three counts. It may take practice.

One of the real benefits of integrating the three-count rhythm into your walks is that it balances the left and right sides of the body. Most people have a dominant foot, just as they have a dominant hand. Often the dominant foot can be determined by looking at wear patterns on your walking shoes. The lead foot, the one that initiates the stride, usually gets the most impact. Not surprisingly, it's also the leg that often shows the first signs of knee problems or foot injuries.

When you consciously choose a three-count walking pattern, both feet get a chance to lead. If you start on the right foot with

In-two-three, then the left foot takes the lead on *OUT-two-three*. If your mind wanders off, you may find yourself counting to three but walking to four: *In-two-three-pause, Out-two-three-pause.* Pay attention, and when you realize you have lost the rhythm, bring yourself back to the three-count. If you haven't already guessed, three-count is the rhythm of a waltz.

2. MENTAL MARINADES: HERE/STRONG

For a variation on the three-step, replace the numbers with words. As you inhale, mentally tell yourself: *I am here.* Three words and three steps per inhalation. As you exhale, mentally say, *I am strong.* Make a chant out of the phrase, repeating, *I am here, I am strong. I am here, I am strong.* And remember to breathe! By saying to yourself, *I am here,* you're affirming that you're present, right now. Your body's here and your mind is also. Not wandering off to gnaw on a problem. *I am strong* is a statement about character, willpower, determination, resourcefulness. It says you're willing and able to maintain focus. Willing and able to follow through with an exercise program. Strong enough to find a way around obstacles in your path—on the walk and in your life. It's a powerful message to give yourself.

3. CHANGE THE MARINADE

Experiment with variations on the words you repeat in a three-beat cadence as you walk. Begin by trying out these phrases:

> I am here, I am calm.
> I am here, I am loved.
> I am here, I am safe.
> I am here, I have faith.
> I am here, life is good.

Sample them all to see how the words feel to you. Each phrase affirms a condition that is true for you in this moment. Right now, I am here. Right now, I am safe. At this time, on this walk. Just for now: *I am here, I am calm.* It doesn't mean that you never feel fear, or never lose faith, or never feel completely, totally alone in the world. Yes, those feelings are true. That is part of who you are. But what about the other parts of you? What about the parts you want to support, strengthen, and have ready to call on when you need them? That's what you affirm when you tell yourself, *I am calm, I am strong, I am loved.*

It takes more than one marinade to keep the menu interesting in the kitchen, and more than one mental marinade to satisfy the appetites of your mind. Some days you may need the "calm" marinade. On others you want the reassurance of "safe" or "strong." Sometimes you may be hungry for "love." You can choose. Try different words for different results.

Previous Exercises You'll Use This Week

As you acquire additional focusing techniques, the mindfulness options available for you on walks are expanding. The walk guidelines below include old as well as new tools. Look back at descriptions in the Walking Well sections of Week One and Week Two if you want to refresh your memory. It may be helpful to jot down an outline of the walk to carry with you.

1. BREATHE IN, BREATHE OUT (WEEK ONE)

Mentally remind yourself *In* as you inhale and *Out* as you exhale. Focusing awareness on the words and breath speeds the release of stress.

2. FOUR-STEP: IN-2-3-4 CADENCE (WEEK TWO)

When you have experimented with the three-step pattern for two or three days, it's interesting to return to the four-count (*In-two-three-four, Out-two-three-four*). Notice the difference in the two walking rhythms. You may prefer one or the other, but using both brings variety to your walks.

3. YIN-YANG BREATH: EARTH AND SKY (WEEK TWO)

A variation on the four-step cadence: Inhale four counts and exhale four counts. As you inhale, imagine drawing yin energy up from the earth, the spirit of receptivity and openness. As you exhale, imagine drawing down the yang energy of the sky, energy of action, and movement.

4. SAY THANK YOU (WEEK ONE)

A moment of appreciation for feet, legs, arms, trees, friends, a warm jacket. Just notice and give thanks. Maintain cadence with "I give thanks" (three-count) or "I am thank-ful" (four-count).

Week Three Goals Overview

Walk Level	Walk Time Goal	Silent Segment Time Goal
Stepping Out	Walk 6 days 12–15 min. a day	10 min. silent
Mid-Stride	Walk 6 days 20 min. 4 days 25 min. 2 days	15–20 min. silent
Strong and Steady	Walk 6 days 30 min. 4–5 days 40 min. 1–2 days	20–30 min. silent

Week Three Daily Walk Guidelines

Rotate walks at your level for variety during the week. Try walks at a different level if you want more or less exercise. Extend any walk by repeating or adding time to a focusing technique. Adjust suggested times to meet personal goals.

Stepping Out		
Week 3	Focusing Techniques Rotate routines for variety	Suggested Timing
3 days 12–15 min.	1. Breathe In, Breathe Out 2. Three-Step: In-2-3 Cadence 3. Yin-Yang Breath: Earth and Sky 4. Say Thank You	5 min. 5 min. 3 min. 2 min.
3 days 12–15 min.	1. Three-Step: In-2-3 Cadence 2. Mental Marinade: Here/Strong 3. Change the Marinade: Variations 4. Say Thank You	3 min. 5 min. 5 min. 2 min.

Mid-Stride		
Week 3	Focusing Techniques Rotate routines for variety	Suggested Timing
4 days 20 min.	1. Breathe In, Breathe Out Or: Walk, Talk, Listen 2. Three-Step: In-2-3 Cadence 3. Mental Marinade: Here/Strong 4. Say Thank You	5 min. 8 min. 5 min. 2 min.
2 days 25 min.	1. Four-Step: In-2-3-4 Cadence Or: Walk, Talk, Listen 2. Yin-Yang Breath: Earth and Sky 3. Three-Step: In-2-3 Cadence 4. Change the Marinade: Variations 5. Say Thank You	8 min. 5 min. 5 min. 5 min. 2 min.

Strong and Steady		
Week 3	Focusing Techniques Rotate routines for variety	Suggested Timing
4–5 days 30 min.	1. Breathe In, Breathe Out Or: Walk, Talk, Listen 2. Three-Step: In-2-3 Cadence 3. Mental Marinade: Here/Strong 4. Change the Marinade: Variations 5. Say Thank You	10 min. 5 min. 5 min. 8 min. 2 min.
1–2 days 40 min.	1. Three-Step: In-2-3 Cadence Or: Walk, Talk, Listen 2. Mental Marinade: Here/Strong 3. Four-Step: In-2-3-4 Cadence 4. Yin-Yang Breath: Earth and Sky 5. Say Thank You	10 min. 10 min. 10 min. 8 min. 2 min.

Log In

Support yourself in maintaining a walking habit by keeping a record of your walks this week in the Week Three Log in the appendix. What was your mood and energy level each day? Did it change after your walk? Did you miss a day? Make a note about what interfered with your schedule. Jot down your response to focusing techniques you are trying this week.

- What did you notice about the three-step cadence of breath, steps, and words? How does it differ from the four-step for you?
- How did it feel to give yourself a positive marinade?
- What words were most significant to you as a useful marinade?
- Did you notice anything on a walk that surprised you or made you smile?

Week Four

A Healthy Self-Image

Imagination can be a creative source of healing. Beliefs and behaviors begin in the mind before they motivate action. Exercise your imagination this week as you add visual imagery to your walks. You'll enhance the benefits of your steps with a mental technique used in athletics, meditation, and healing.

*B*y the fourth month of chemotherapy, my closet held an assortment of wigs. One of them offered the reassurance of familiarity—a well-behaved pageboy that mirrored the hair I'd worn before breast cancer treatment. Others dressed me in new identities. Some days I chose a curly mophead that mushroomed around my face. On others, I emerged as a trendy barista with hair of flaming magenta. The variety helped lighten the harsh reality of cancer. Bewigged I felt almost costumed, as if I could don a new reality and step away from the fears exposed by a bald scalp.

But when I decided to walk in the Susan G. Komen Foundation Race for the Cure, I went shopping for new headgear. I wanted a pink bandana for my head. Just enough coverage to temper reality, but not to disguise my situation. This wasn't the first time I had joined participants in a cancer fundraising walk, but it was the first time I lined up in a pink tee shirt—the badge of a cancer patient instead of a supporter. The difference is enormous. Huddled in a crowd of 10,000 survivors and supporters, I felt trapped in an identity that bewildered me. On every side, I confronted the presence of pink—a strong and stunning visual proclamation of cancer's impact.

"How ya' doing?" a voice beside me asked. A pink-shirted woman draped an arm loosely around my shoulder as I stepped into the swell of bodies moving toward the starting line. I felt my throat tighten with emotion. "I don't know," I stammered. "I'm pretty new at this."

"Ah, you'll be fine," the stranger promised. "Look at us." Her free arm swept to a group of laughing women whose voices resonated with friendship and vitality. They all had hair. They all looked strong. "We're all survivors and so are you," she said. "You're a survivor, too."

When she moved forward to join her group of friends, my eyes followed the words printed on the back of the pink tee shirt she wore. "I will survive. I have so much life to live. I have so much love to give," proclaimed the message stamped on the pink shirts surrounding me. The words lodged in the tightness of my throat. I wore the same words on the back of my shirt but the fit felt pretentious and hollow.

"Survivor" felt like wishful thinking at this stage of my cancer experience. How could a cancer patient be called a survivor? I'd already stumbled on the word once in this walk. The registration form had asked me to identify myself by checking either "survivor" or "supporter" on the form. I responded with indignation. As an active cancer patient, I felt excluded from either category. My friend Pat had gently set me straight. She'd faced the fears of cancer one year before me. "OK," she said patiently, after listening to my protests. "Here's the question: Are you alive today?" She paused and waited for the words to penetrate my resistance. "That's all there is," she counseled. "That's all there ever is. If you're alive today, then today you're a survivor."

A new definition, a new self-image, settled slowly over me with her words. I allowed myself to imagine stepping away from the limbo of "patient in treatment," which puts life in a temporary stall—on hold until further notice. Still, all those pink shirts rocked my confidence. So many walkers, declaring an intention to survive. So many people living strong amid uncertainty. I wondered if I would ever find enough balance to laugh with my friends and celebrate survival, like the woman who had wrapped a knowing arm around me at the start of the walk.

In the days following the cancer walk, I returned home to the neighborhood walks that gave continuity to my days. My walks were often shorter now, and the pace slower than in the past when fitness walks had pushed me to aerobic levels. My goal had changed. "The best way out is always through," advises a line from a Robert Frost poem. I knew that for me, the best way through a time of stress and challenge is on a walking path.

While I walked the streets of my neighborhood, I carried in my mind an image of the pink shirts pulling me forward. The brash authority of those words both attracted and unnerved me: "I will survive. I have so much life to live. I have so much love to give." With time, the words settled into a phrase that I could believe. They found a rhythm that matched my steps: *Here and now, I'm a-live. Here and now, I sur-vive.* I walked with the words flowing in cadence with my steps, forming a prayer and an affirmation.

As I moved through chemotherapy and radiation and plunged into the gaping uncertainty that marks the end of treatment, I clutched the calming mantra. *Here and now, I'm a-live. Here and now, I sur-vive.* Gradually, my steps brought me closer to acceptance. I felt my confidence shift. Instead of waiting for confirmation of a cure, I edged toward reconciliation with the identity of a survivor, learning to live with the shadows. Then, six months after completion of treatment, I rounded the corner on a morning hike and met the sun rising up to meet me face-to-face. Radiant light enveloped me and in an instant, I felt warm again, trusting the cycle of life that begins anew day after day. Bathed in the sun, I found the courage to stop waiting for a blood test or an accumulation of sufficient years to assure me I could finally embrace the status of survivor. *Here and now, I'm a-live.*

Everyday Survival

No matter how often we tell ourselves that life is an uncertain proposition and that there are no guarantees for any of us, most of the time we live with the belief that what doesn't get done today can wait until tomorrow. When a crisis cracks our faith in tomorrow, we are reminded that nothing is certain. It is a condition of human life that we all encounter events or illnesses that shatter assumptions. These high-stress situations shake more than our mental expectations; they upset the harmony of our biological systems. Research consistently demonstrates the dramatic role of stress in accelerating the risk of illness and pain. Survival requires recognition of both physical and emotional aspects of healing.

It is quite possible to emerge physically from the trauma of a heart attack, or a divorce, or the violence of war, but not to survive emotionally. We all know people who seem caught inside the identity of victim, unable to achieve the healing that allows one to move on. They may be cured physically, but they are not healed.

Emotional healing began with accepting the crucial differences between "cured" and "healed."

When I entered medical treatment for metastatic cancer, the course of my physical healing began. Emotional healing lagged behind. It began when I stepped into a healthy self-image that shifted my focus from "what if" to "what is." It began when I learned to accept the crucial differences between "cured" and "healed." By pulling the words apart, my vocabulary expanded, and so did my options. Healthy, I decided, is largely a mental and emotional state, an attitude. It isn't dependent on "cure." Right now, I am a strong and healthy survivor.

Rather than live in fear of the unknown, I chose to put more weight on what was known—I feel strong and healthy and full of life. Instead of focusing on the fact that no test could prove my body was cancer free, even after treatment, I made an effort to focus on today. At this moment, my body is symptom-free. It isn't simply mind over matter; it's a cooperative agreement of mind *and* matter. Yes, my body still registers icy fear when I learn of a friend's reoccurrence. I don't deny the vulnerability I feel when I report for a mammogram. There is room in my mind for both fear and faith. "I am large, I contain multitudes," as Walt Whitman proclaimed in his epic poem "Song of Myself."

Say Yes Quickly

Language reflects these polar points of view. To define "survivor" as an identity that requires a *guarantee* of health puts the focus on what could still go wrong. To define "survivor" as meaning that today, at least, I have outlived the risk, turns attention to what is going right in this moment. I have a choice about which position to take in defining my life. It isn't always an easy choice, even for a person who loves the complexity of words. As a writer and former newspaper journalist, I delight in words. But it wasn't writing that taught me full appreciation for the role of language in shaping imagination. I was in my mid-forties before I discovered that words are implements of health and self-acceptance. When enthusiasm for walking carried me into competitive racewalking, I experienced the power of words to mold a new self-image and transform a physical klutz into a successful athlete.

For years, I had defined myself as a "klutz," putting my focus on every stumble, bump, and misstep that I took. If I hoped to succeed as a competitive racewalker, I had to change my language. To redirect my focus, I created an affirmation that I wrote daily in my journal and often repeated mentally as I walked: *I am a graceful and active woman, at ease in a strong, healthy body.* The words portrayed an image that I didn't really trust. At first they felt awkward and untrue. But they described how I wanted to feel in my body—at ease and safe.

Gradually, the words planted themselves in my mind and in my personal beliefs. They became the truth about how I felt and how I viewed myself. Then a cancer diagnosis shattered the relationship I had established with my body. Unable to call myself a "healthy woman," I didn't know who I was.

I suspect a similar jolt to self-image occurs when the change is from wife to widow. Or from husband to divorced male. From business professional to stroke victim. From diabetic to amputee. From homeowner to homeless hurricane victim. Trauma often upsets identity and demands a revised self-definition. When you can pair your steps with words or images that dispel your loss of stability or identity, you speed the healing process. Even a moment or two of tranquility allows the cells to stop tensing for attack and begin movement toward recovery. When I repeated the phrase *I'm a-live, I sur-vive* as I walked, the words created a three-count cadence with my steps that helped sustain momentum and energy. But more importantly, the chant stopped the cycle of worry and doubt that dominated my mind otherwise. Gradually, the words helped shift my mental picture of myself from victim to victor.

The power of mental pictures to influence healing, well-being, self-image, and performance is widely recognized in athletics, health care, and psychology. We all carry internal portraits that help or hinder us as we move through life. These fantasy images, researchers say, guide behavior and choices. The pictures we see of ourselves in the future—in situations that can be either positive or negative—are termed "possible selves" by psychologists.

The ability to imagine oneself going to college someday can motivate a middle school student to make wise choices in completing homework, for example. The ability to see oneself attending the distant wedding of a grandchild can give a diabetic incentive to remain active and mindful of healthy choices. The ability to visualize oneself hiking the Appalachian Trail can strengthen a heart disease survivor's commitment to exercise and diet.

Research at Oregon State University suggests that our ability to imagine a positive future for ourselves through "possible selves" bolsters our ability to weather the challenges of aging and the upheaval of illness, transitions, and life events. The findings support the words of a popular motivational quote from educator William Arthur Ward: "If you can imagine it, you can achieve it; if you can dream it, you can become it."

In Her Wildest Dreams

In her wildest dreams, Tammey Burns saw herself gliding the length of a swimming pool with a strong and steady stroke. She toed the starting line at track meets and felt the energy of an athlete coursing through her veins. In her wildest dreams, she was sleek and fast—an active participant in life. But that was only in her dreams. In the light of day, she retreated to the sidelines and comforted herself with food.

"Ever since I was little, I was an athlete wanna-be, but I never thought I was good enough or thin enough or disciplined enough," she says.[1] "I struggled with weight all my life. I was pretty much the wallflower, and food was my drug of choice. Food was a friend. It didn't talk back to me, so I didn't have to deal with emotional issues."

By the time Tammey reached forty, obesity smothered even her dreams. When her weight hit 575 pounds, the only "possible self" she could imagine was life as an invalid. Standing for more than a couple minutes caused severe pain in her hips and back. She could walk no more than two or three steps. She couldn't get into a car, fit into a theater seat, lift herself up a single stair step, or attend to her personal hygiene. Squeezing her massive body into the shower at home was almost impossible. She had been diagnosed with twelve weight-related medical problems, including diabetes, hypertension, sleep apnea, restrictive lung disease, obesity hypoventilation syndrome, and venous stasis insufficiency. The right side of her enlarged heart was failing. Day and night, she was tethered to a tank that dispensed five liters of oxygen daily.

"I felt hopeless and helpless and useless," she says. "I hated myself and what I had let myself become." It took a failed attempt at suicide to shape a new self-image. If God wanted her alive, she decided, she had better get ready for what life might bring next. She began to ponder a new "possible self"—one that could face the world without an addiction to food. The vision pulled her through dieting, counseling, soul searching, and gym workouts. Then it brought her back to an adolescent dream. Once again, she envisions herself as an athlete. Seven years after her suicide attempt and down more than 400 pounds, she is training to walk thirteen miles in a half marathon.

"I'm no longer the fat girl on the sidelines. I'm an athlete," she exclaims. The transformation has been long and strenuous. "Self-image is a huge issue that I have had to change. I was fat and ugly. I know what it is like to try to commit suicide. Now, I'm in better health than I have ever been. It's been a slow process, but it has been an amazing journey."

A graduate of Missouri State University with a degree in recreation therapy, Tammey worked as an activities director in Springfield, Missouri, nursing homes before weight and health confined her to a sedentary life in the house shared with her mother and sister. Four years after her suicide attempt, she had managed to drop more than 170 pounds by dieting. She held a desk job with an insurance company. But at 403 pounds, her body continued to balk at the load. Supplemental oxygen no longer sustained her adequately, and doctors implanted a tracheotomy tube in her throat to provide a direct line of air into her lungs. The tube would be permanent, they told her, unless she could lose 120 pounds more.

"I wanted the tube out," she says. "I knew I had to quit fad diets and work on the emotional issues to find out why I had such a strong addiction to food. I knew I had to start working from the inside out." When she found a magazine picture of a woman who weighed 150 pounds, she cut it out and pasted a photo of her own face on the body. Below the picture she wrote the line that fueled commitment and fostered a new self-image: "A journey of a thousand miles begins with one step."

A year later, with her weight down to 355, she added exercise to her weight-loss regimen. When she joined the fitness center at a local hospital, people stared. Some laughed. But six days a week, she showed up at 5:30 AM, knowing that she had to schedule workouts before job, family, or church activities muddied her commitment to change. With a tracheotomy hole in her throat, she could not swim, but she wanted the buoyancy of water. She started with fifteen minutes of water walking in the medical center's four-foot-deep therapy pool. When she had built up enough endurance to walk the pool for thirty minutes, she branched out to an exercise bike. Four months later, she ventured onto the workout track and walked a lap, one-tenth of a mile. That's when she met Colleen Young, mind-body fitness coordinator at the gym and a competitive racewalker. Colleen had been watching Tammey's efforts. She recognized a gritty determination that an oversize body could not hide. When she offered to coach Tammey in a walking program, the suggestion shocked and fascinated the overweight woman.

"When Colleen said she wanted to work with me, I thought, What does this woman see?" recalls Tammey. "I was over 300 pounds! She came along at a time when nobody else believed in me. Even I didn't believe in myself. But God let her see my potential, and it has been an amazing journey."

At a weight of 303 pounds and a bandage collar protecting the trach hole in her throat, Tammey walked a five-kilometer community walk with Colleen at her side, coaching, prodding, and encouraging. One year later, with her weight down to 198 and the tracheostomy closed, she completed a ten-kilometer walk, and knew that she was hooked. A new dream took shape in her mind. "I want to be a nationally ranked competitive racewalker," she says, "At first, it was a lot of work, but I just couldn't believe there was something that could be this much fun. When those endorphins get flowing, it's such a high."

"If you get the spirit moving, the body will follow."

The turning point in her health and in her zest for life, she says, came when she started focusing on the inside rather than the outside. With guidance from Colleen, she turned the goal to fitness rather than weight loss. She aimed at making her body dynamic and strong, shifting emphasis from appearance to performance. Food became fuel to give her energy and endurance as an athlete, rather than a source of comfort and consolation. Eight years after she tried to end her life, Tammey's weight has dropped to 165 on the way to a goal of 150. She has been cleared of nine serious medical conditions. Diet and exercise now control her diabetes.

"My success isn't simply that I have lost this incredible amount of weight, or that I have never failed. My success is that I have gotten up one more time to try again," she says. "There is no magic pill. It takes a lot of determination and commitment. Attitude is everything."

At the gym, the laughing has stopped, her coach says. When people stare these days, it is with respect. "Tammey learned how to connect with her inner self, not to see herself as ugly," says Colleen Young.[2] "If you get the spirit moving, the body will follow. That's the premise I use with everyone."

Now Tammey likes to visualize her transformational journey as parallel to the annual flight of monarch butterflies who wing south from the United States each fall to winter on a hilltop in Mexico. Their trip is long, she says, and certainly there are challenges that might push the butterflies off course. Winds, rains, birds—any number of interferences to navigate. But instinct drives the monarchs to focus on the goal, not on the struggle. "That's what I do," she says. "I celebrate the little wins along the way, but I focus on the long term. The statistics for morbidly obese people to lose weight and keep it off are very small. You have to work from within."

In addition to maintaining a six-day-a-week exercise schedule in preparation for her first half marathon, Tammey is working on certification with the American College of Sports Medicine as a personal trainer and wellness coach. "I cannot imagine returning to my former, dismal self," she says. "Life is such an amazing adventure, if you let it be."

SIDE STEPS: *Walking and Muscles*

Skeletal muscles make up the largest tissue component of the human body, accounting for about 40 percent of your weight. Strong muscles protect you against injury. They're essential for balance, mobility, and physical vitality. When illness, accidents, and emotional upheaval take you out of action, muscle loss becomes another side effect, and another facet of healing. Even a few days of inactivity results in significant muscle atrophy.

Astronauts confined to the weightlessness of space return to Earth with weaker muscles. Young people who are bedridden experience loss of muscle strength similar to that seen in the aging process. Age-related decline in muscle mass and function is called sarcopenia and is part of normal aging, but inactivity is a serious contributor. By age eighty, most people will have lost 30 to 40 percent of their peak strength.[3]

Muscle cells burn calories more efficiently than fat cells, so when you lose muscle, you may experience weight gain. As muscle mass declines, fat cells move in, contributing to belly fat and flabby thighs. And because your muscles provide a storehouse for blood sugar, the loss of muscle results in higher blood sugar, which elevates the risk of type-2 diabetes.

Fortunately, with regular exercise and strength training, it is possible to rebuild muscle. As you enter the fourth week of this walking program, you may be feeling stronger already. As a rule of thumb, it takes about three weeks for the body to adjust to the demands of a new level of exercise.[4] Walking triggers movement in many muscle groups and provides a good base for improved strength and flexibility. But a combination of aerobic exercise and weight training is recommended for maximum muscle health at any age.

STEP IT UP

If you are physically ready to boost the weight-bearing workout you get from a walk, try adding a stairway to your route. Or step up and down on the curb a few times at the end of the walk, when your muscles are warmed up. Lifting your body weight up a step or curb will build strength in the quadriceps muscles on the front of the thighs, decreasing stress on the knees and reducing arthritis pain.

WEIGHT IT OUT

When you add weight training to your exercise program, make it separate from your walks. The use of hand or ankle weights while walking can interfere with posture and contribute to injuries. Instead, consider using the equipment at a fitness center. In studies at Tufts University, men who exercised three times a week for twelve weeks on a machine designed to build thigh muscles increased strength in muscles that bend the knee joint 226 percent.[5]

STRETCH IT OUT

Depending on the level of the walks you are following, you may want to give your muscles both a warm-up and warm-down phase. Often this happens naturally. Just two or three minutes of leisurely walking can boost circulation and oxygen flow to your muscles at the start of a walk, preparing you for a more active pace.

To keep your muscles moving smoothly, take time for a few simple stretches at the conclusion of a walk. Do your stretches after walking, when muscles are warm, rather than before you start. If you feel stiff at the beginning of a walk, loosen up by rotating each foot at the ankle a few times. Circle your hips, and do some shoulder rolls to gently release the joints. At the end of the walk, repeat those rotations. Now is the time to add in some leg stretches to loosen calf and thigh muscles. Say thanks to your muscles as you stretch.

*The real voyage of discovery consists not in seeking
new landscapes, but in having new eyes.*

—Marcel Proust

When you imagine yourself in a setting you love, a place where you feel safe and at peace, blood pressure drops, heart rate slows, and breathing becomes deeper. Where the mind goes, energy or life force follows. It is a powerful, cooperative relationship.

That relationship comes into play when we think about self-image. "Image" and "imagination" come from the same old Latin root, *imago*. Yet, when it comes to self-image, we often curb imagination. We forget that change begins in the mind, and get stuck in an image that seems set and inflexible. Sometimes it takes a crisis to reignite the fires of creativity that give us new eyes.

A diagnosis of osteoporosis following my cancer treatment—bone loss accelerated by chemotherapy—triggered an image of tottering frailty. In my mind, it painted me as stooped and fragile, slowed by disease. The image terrified me. Then it motivated me to make strength training a more consistent component of my exercise program. Gradually, my image rebounded—no longer frail, but strong and determined, living with awareness and action.

Last week, the focusing techniques you used on walks emphasized the power of words to assist you in releasing stress and reaffirming goals. This week, the exercises encourage you to free your imagination as you continue to explore techniques of focus that are shared by athletes and meditators: breath awareness, words and self-talk, visual imagery, and practice.

Some people find that words can be distracting, sending the mind off on chains of thought. If that happened for you, this week's focus on visual images offers an alternative. It's not necessary to create a mental picture to use visualization. Many people find it difficult to "see" an image mentally. You need only suggest an image to your brain and then imagine the feeling it produces. You've already used imagery to smooth out your step when you visualize your foot as a rocker in the Put Your Foot Down exercise. This week, practice mental images that support your posture and your energy.

1. STRONG AND SMOOTH IMAGE

This three-count exercise combines two focusing techniques that you practiced in previous weeks. Last week, you created a three-beat cadence that combined breath, steps, and words. This week, continue that formula, but add a visual image from Week One that helps you maintain a smooth stride. The vision of your foot as a rocker, like the bottom of a rocking chair, gives you a picture that guides you in using your entire foot for each step, rolling from the heel to the toe. This stride reduces impact and improves posture as you walk.

Mentally, repeat to yourself *I am strong, I am smooth,* as you establish a three-count cadence. Inhale for three steps and exhale for three steps. As you hear *smooth* in your mind, imagine that your foot is a rocker, gliding along the path without shuffling or slapping the ground. When you hear *strong* in your mind, imagine your body moving with ease and agility. Strong and smooth. The words provide reminders, and visual images, that help you focus on posture.

2. SMOOTH AND TALL IMAGE

This exercise is a useful variation on the previous three-count. It adds a visual picture that helps you maintain tall, stable posture as you walk. Imagine that you have a cable attached to the top of your head that connects to a kind of trolley line overhead. The trolley line lifts your body gently, and also provides energy that draws you forward. Some people can actually "see" a cable in their mind's eye. Some people simply "feel" the pull of a cable stretching up from the top of the head to gently lift the torso. Now combine the cable with the rocker on your feet. (Remember, your brain will find ways to entertain itself if you don't give it variety. Be playful and let your mind enjoy the game.)

Mentally tell yourself, *I am smooth, I am tall.* Maintain the cadence with three words and three steps each for inhalation and exhalation. Use your creative imagination to "see" or "feel" the cable holding you upright as you say *tall.* Imagine a rolling rocker on the bottom of your foot when you say *smooth.* This is a wonderful technique for restoring good posture and opening your lungs for full breathing anytime you begin to feel bogged down and weary on a walk.

3. LOVE IN, FEAR OUT

As the quote that introduces this section suggests, when you can't change the landscape, perhaps you can change your perspective or shift your point of view. That's what this exercise helps you do. It uses the power of words and imagination to open your heart and to refocus your thoughts.

Continue using the three-count cadence for this exercise, changing the words so that when you inhale, you mentally say, *Love comes in.* When you exhale, say, *Fear goes out.* Add your own imagination to the formula by thinking of love coming into you as you inhale. Try to imagine love flowing up from the ground, or from the air, or the landscape around you. Feel love filling your lungs and your heart. As you exhale, think of flushing fear out of your cells. Let it evaporate into thin air. Feel the space left in your lungs when fear is released. Then inhale love again. Maintain the three-count rhythm by repeating, *Love comes in, Fear goes out.*

In times of severe stress, fear dominates our minds and emotions. People around us may offer love, but it's hard to let that in. I began doing this visual exercise during chemotherapy treatment, at a time when many people were sincerely concerned about my well-being. I was so filled with fear and dread that I was unable to accept their love. I cringed internally when people tried to reassure or comfort me. I feared I would crack if I relaxed. But I wanted love. To confront the emotional conflict

I was feeling, I practiced breathing in love and breathing out fear as part of my daily walks. Words and breath began to open me to trust, and then to love.

4. BUNGEE CORD

A healthy imagination is a great resource when you begin to extend the length of your walks or when you are tempted to cut a walk short. Just use your mind to create a bungee cord that keeps you moving toward your goal! Try this exercise on a straight stretch of your walk route—someplace where you have street signs, light posts, mailboxes, or trees at regular intervals. Imagine that you have a hefty bungee cord—the kind that people use to jump off bridges. Loop one end around your hips. Imagine that you can feel it snug on your hips. Hook the other end of the bungee to a telephone pole, light post, tree, or mailbox ahead of you on your path. (Play along here—this is imagination!) Keep your eye on the post and start walking. Feel the energy of the bungee cord pulling you forward as you maintain focus on your target. When you get close to the end of your cord, look ahead and hook it to the next target along the path. Post by post, tree by tree, you move smoothly ahead, letting the cord pull you. Each post becomes a goal achieved. Each segment, a new conquest. It's a mental game that keeps motivation fresh, and it's also a convincing metaphor for the power of keeping your eye on your goal. In addition to energizing your walk, the practice of focusing on a point ahead of you as you walk helps you maintain a good, upright walking posture.

Previous Exercises You'll Use This Week

1. BREATHE IN, BREATHE OUT (WEEK ONE)

Mentally remind yourself *In* as you inhale and *Out* as you exhale. Focusing awareness on the words and breath speeds the release of stress.

2. PUT YOUR FOOT DOWN (WEEK ONE)

Imagine your foot is a rocker, rolling smoothly along the ground with each step. Feel the solid footing beneath you. Notice your stability.

3. CHANGE THE MARINADE (WEEK THREE)

Free your creative chi to assist you in shaping a three-beat marinade that affirms a condition you want to validate or reinforce in your life. Perhaps you found a word last week that reverberated in your soul. Use it again this week to infuse your cells with a healing marinade. Already this week, you've used a form of mental marinade as you repeat *I am strong, I am smooth, I am tall.* Change the marinade with words that have significance to you. *I am calm, I am loved, I am safe,* for example.

4. YIN-YANG BREATH: EARTH AND SKY (WEEK TWO)

As you inhale, imagine drawing yin energy up from the earth, the spirit of receptivity and openness. As you exhale, imagine drawing down the yang energy of the sky, energy of action and movement. Use either three- or four-count cadence.

5. SAY THANK YOU (WEEK ONE)

Thank your feet, your hips, and your imagination. Give thanks for sunshine or for rain. Maintain cadence with *I give thanks* (three-count) or *I am thank-ful* (four-count).

Week Four Goals Overview

Walk Level	Walk Time Goal	Silent Segment Time Goal
Stepping Out	Walk 6 days 14–16 min. a day	10 min. silent
Mid-Stride	Walk 6 days 20 min. 3 days 25 min. 3 days	15–20 min. silent
Strong and Steady	Walk 6 days 30 min. 4–5 days 40 min. 1–2 days	20–30 min. silent

Week Four Daily Walk Guidelines

Rotate walks at your level for variety during the week. Try walks at a different level if you want more or less exercise. Extend walks if you wish by repeating or adding time to a focusing technique. Adjust suggested timing to meet your personal goals.

Stepping Out		
Week 4	**Focusing Techniques** Rotate routines for variety	**Suggested Timing**
2 days 14–16 min.	1. Breathe In, Breathe Out	4 min.
	2. Strong and Smooth: In-2-3 Cadence	5 min.
	3. Smooth and Tall: In-2-3 Cadence	5 min.
	4. Say Thank You	2 min.
2 days 14–16 min.	1. Strong and Smooth: In-2-3 Cadence	5 min.
	2. Change the Marinade: Three-Count Cadence	5 min.
	3. Bungee Cord	4 min.
	4. Say Thank You	2 min.

(continued on the next page)

Stepping Out		
Week 4	Focusing Techniques Rotate routines for variety	Suggested Timing
2 days 14–16 min.	1. Put Your Foot Down 2. Yin-Yang Breath: Earth and Sky 3. Love In, Fear Out: In-2-3 Cadence 4. Say Thank You	5 min. 4 min. 5 min. 2 min.

Mid-Stride		
Week 4	Focusing Techniques Rotate routines for variety	Suggested Timing

3 days
20 min.
	1. Put Your Foot Down
	   Or: Walk, Talk, Listen
	2. Strong and Smooth: In-2-3
	   Cadence
	3. Smooth and Tall: In-2-3 Cadence
	4. Say Thank You
		5 min.
		
		7 min.
		
		6 min.
		2 min.

3 days
25 min.
	1. Yin-Yang Breath: Earth and Sky
	   Or: Walk, Talk, Listen
	2. Love In, Fear Out: In-2-3 Cadence
	3. Change the Marinade:
	   Three-Count Cadence
	4. Bungee Cord
	5. Say Thank You
		5 min.
		
		5 min.
		8 min.
		
		5 min.
		2 min.

Strong and Steady		
Week 4	Focusing Techniques Rotate routines for variety	Suggested Timing

4–5 days
30 min.
	1. Put Your Foot Down
	   Or: Walk, Talk, Listen
	2. Love In, Fear Out: In-2-3 Cadence
	3. Strong and Smooth:
	   In-2-3 Cadence
	4. Bungee Cord
	5. Say Thank You
		8 min.
		
		5 min.
		5 min.
		
		10 min.
		2 min.

Strong and Steady		
Week 4	Focusing Techniques Rotate routines for variety	Suggested Timing
1–2 days 40 min.	1. Strong and Smooth: In-2-3 Cadence Or: Walk, Talk, Listen	10 min.
	2. Smooth and Tall: In-2-3 Cadence	10 min.
	3. Change the Marinade: Three-Count Cadence	10 min.
	4. Yin-Yang Breath: Earth and Sky	8 min.
	5. Say Thank You	2 min.

Log In

Use the Week Four log in the appendix to record your walks and your experiences this week. Notice your mood, your energy, and your posture at the beginning and end of the walks.

- What do you notice about your posture when you affirm that you are strong and tall? Or tall and smooth?
- Are you comfortable with the *In-2-3* cadence?
- How did it feel to inhale love? To release fear?
- What did you learn about yourself on this walk?
- Did you see something with new eyes on your walk?
- What "marinade" words feel helpful?
- What are you thankful for?

Week Five

A Healthy Rhythm

> Whether the rhythm is a march, a waltz, or a chanted prayer, the cadence created by a blending of words, breath, and steps generates momentum that can carry you through rough spots and weariness. This week, engage your spirit by adding mental music to your walks. Feel your steps lighten, your mood brighten, as rhythm produces a healing wholeness.

W
e were south of the Scottish border, but not far south, when the words of a familiar highlands ballad began to set the pace of my steps. They emerged at the approach to a crossroads on the trail, and at every intersection. "Oh, ye'll take the high road and I'll take the low road, and I'll be in Scotland afore ye."

On the first day of a walking vacation in the Lake District of northern England, we mulled our decisions carefully. Should we take the path that climbed to higher elevations? Or choose the trail that dropped into the valley beside the splashing stream? The trails were unknown, the weather uncertain. We pulled out the guidebook and pondered our choices.

"Go high," I'd urge. "Go low," my spouse would counter. As independent travelers, we had no tour guide to settle the question.

The high road? The low road? We had the freedom to take either path. For ten unscheduled days we could set our own course in exploring the network of trails that lace the Lake District National Park's 855-square-mile area.

Gradually, we settled into the reflective quiet of uninterrupted walking that lay between junctions. Feet and spirit in step with the rhythm of movement. As the hours and the miles dropped behind us, a playful pattern emerged. "Go high," I'd suggest as we approached a trail sign. Then I backed my position with a new twist on the familiar song. "Oh, let's take the high road, the reach-for-the-sky road," I'd sing aloud. Not to be outdone, my husband rose to the challenge. A few turns later, he had a musical proposal of his own: "Oh, let's take the low road, the gentle and slow road," he proposed.

Most of the time, the decision rested not on lyrics but on maps that identified the path most likely to bring us back to our lodging. As we walked, sometimes up and sometimes down, the melody and words became a meditation playing softly at the back of my mind. A lullaby of sorts to gently brush aside thoughts of home and the harder decisions that had preceded this vacation. My mother's death, just one month prior to our long-planned departure date, transformed a holiday into a requiem—a journey of reflection, renewal, and redirection for me.

We had planned the trip as a much-anticipated return to lush green landscapes, to hillsides thick with bracken, to mountain streams, stacked slate fences, and pristine lakes that delighted us a decade earlier when we first visited these trails on England's northern border. The wild beauty that inspired the nineteenth-century Lake Poets had charmed me, as well. I looked forward to vigorous walks and rewarding views.

But life events reshaped the vision. Until four months before her death, at age ninety-seven, my mother lived a fiercely independent life. It took a disabling fall to force her out of the house where she had resided for sixty years and into a care facility. Death brought a form of independence that she did not dread. It brought, for me, freedom from the priorities and patterns of responsibility that often fall to a firstborn child. For months before her death, I traveled an hour up the freeway several times a week to assist with the increasing complications of her life. The bills, the banking, the laundry, and the soothing of complaints about home health providers imposed a regime of caregiving on my days. The losses my mother battled as her body declined made painful demands on both of us. Letting go. Holding on. We alternated positions and struggled for control. Resentment flared when my efforts failed to satisfy. They flipped, on a smile, to gratitude for the opportunity to feel helpful.

Her death carried me headlong into cleaning, sorting, discarding, boxing, and burning sixty years of thrift wedged into every crevice of her home. Bags of buttons, used zippers torn from worn clothing, fabric scraps, outdated calendars, corsage pins, Sunday programs from church—nothing too old or tattered or dated to be saved "in case" it could be used again. From the attic to the garage, the dust of history enveloped me as I sorted trash and treasures, unearthing landmarks and landmines from her past, and from my own.

By the time I locked the door of her hushed, half-emptied home and boarded the airplane, I was exhausted. The serendipity of an extended walking trip one month after this upheaval in my life seemed almost a miracle. I longed for the quiet comfort of nature and for the steady cadence of walks that restore balance and clarity. For the first time in several years, I could head off on a trip without the nagging awareness that any phone call might be a summons home. This time, my mother traveled with me.

The outing couldn't have come at a more perfect time to soothe the emotional storms I'd encountered. The weather that greeted our arrival in England was another matter. Rain splashed the windows of the taxi that delivered us from the train station at Oxenholme to a small hotel on the banks of Grasmere Lake. Streams of water dulled the view from our hotel room, across a pasture of newly sheared sheep, down to a gray, sullen lake. We unpacked boots, umbrellas, and raincoats and rued the decision to leave behind waterproof Gortex pants. We fell asleep with the sounds of rain in our ears and awoke to the same score.

William Wordsworth, writing about the Lake District weather in his 1835 *Guide to the Lakes,* says, "Days of unsettled weather, with partial showers, are very frequent; but the showers, darkening, or brightening, as they fly from hill to hill, are not less grateful to the eye than finely interwoven passages of gay and sad music are touching to the ear."[1]

Alas, the sound of rain was not the refrain I wanted to hear on the first morning of a walking vacation. I groused and grumbled and complained. I sulked and sipped another cup of tea. Trails we'd planned to walk would be slick and uninviting, the views obscured by clouds. Although I didn't realize it then, I'd encountered the first crossroads of this journey—a chance to take the high road or the low. As commonly used, the phrase "take the high road" implies choosing the moral, ethical path—to do the right thing. It is not an easy path. It demands that you make an uphill push through the initial disappointment, fear, discomfort, inconvenience, outrage, pain, or grief that stops you at a decision point.

That first morning in the Lake District, all I could see was a dead end. By noon, the clouds began to thin along the flanks of nearby hills. The gray ceiling brightened just enough to suggest the possibility of a dry afternoon. It was all the encouragement we needed. We set out with a goal of walking to a neighboring village along a low path that skirted the lake and climbed a gentle slope with views of the country house where Wordsworth once lived. By the time we'd rounded the lake, a spit of rain dampened the guidebook that we carried. We tucked it into a daypack and kept walking, letting trail markers and common sense guide us to the village and safely back.

In the days ahead, we journeyed past resistance to resignation in daily confrontations with the weather. The perfect timing of our trip coincided with one of the wettest summers on record in Western Europe. County councils cancelled local fairs due to standing water in playing fields. Weddings booked for the shores of pristine lakes took refuge in crowded hotel parlors. Mountain rivulets became rushing streams to be crossed, hopscotch style, on stones. Everywhere we encountered the impact of rain and the junction of decision.

Shrouded in green plastic ponchos, we sloshed along trails running with water and gave thanks for waterproof boots. We traversed boggy wetlands on the summits and tramped through mud at the edge of streams. Day after day, I waited for grief to splash more moisture on my path. Without the tasks of transition to distract me, I expected sorrow to catch me as the rhythm of my pace slowed. Instead I encountered a void. Bereft of the matriarchal force I had leaned into or pushed against for my entire life, vast emptiness opened before me. I plodded forward blindly into a life cut loose from the family framework that had shaped me. Overhead the sky sobbed as I skirted the unknown. High road? Low road? It didn't matter. Both guided me toward balance, aware of the bloodline revealed in my own steps. The character trait I'd labeled "stubbornness" in my mother, I dubbed "determination" in myself.

Legend says the Scottish ballad that brought lightness to our steps was initially a song of grief—the farewell lament of a dying soldier to his sweetheart. In our application, it didn't feel like a dirge at all. It felt like an anthem to options—to choices, decisions, farewells, and fresh steps. It consoled and coached like a gentle reminder to choose the high road as I crossed the chasm of motherlessness.

Take the High Road

All of us encounter crossroads in life. In times of upheaval, decisions seem to stack up before us, leaving no space for recovery in between. It may help, in these moments, to "take the high road," literally, when making a decision. Get on your feet and take a walk. Just get moving and you'll be on a path that leads to a change of position and perspective that may be more than physical.

When emotion blocks your view of the choices ahead, it's a natural response to withdraw and hope that the storm will pass.

But the high road calls for positive steps. It urges you to pause long enough to check your map. Where will each choice take you? What is the outcome that leads to the greatest good or satisfaction? The least pain?

Take the high road when making a decision—take a walk before taking action.

It may have been stubbornness that propelled me to hike in spite of the weather on the first days of our trip. But gradually the path led to the destination I was seeking—not physical landmarks but spiritual ones. What cleared was not the sky but my outlook. Movement restored my balance, physically and emotionally. It left me better prepared to shape my future, as well as sort through legal and family issues that I inherited with my mother's passing.

Walking does more than get your feet back on the ground or help you catch a breath of fresh air. The rhythmic side-to-side movement of walking actually benefits your brain. Bilateral movement in which both sides of the body work in tandem, as in walking, swimming, or running, sends impulses to both the left and right hemispheres of the brain, activating resources of the whole brain. Research in child development and in adult recovery from stroke has demonstrated the effectiveness of bilateral movement in creating or restoring healthy brain patterns.

If rhythmic, repetitive bilateral movement helps repattern the brains of stroke victims, doesn't it seem possible that walking might facilitate the repatterning of some of your own nonproductive mental paths? Andrew Weil, physician, author, and outspoken advocate of natural healing processes, is an enthusiastic walker. Weil credits bilateral movement, in which the right leg and left arm move forward at the same time, then the left leg and the right arm move together, with creating a "harmonizing influence on the whole central nervous system."[2] Without the resourcefulness of both hemispheres of the brain, it's more difficult to heal from emotional stresses and more difficult to make clear, wise choices. We get stuck in one-channel thinking that limits options.

The action of getting started on a walk almost always begins at a crossroads of choice. Maybe it's the weather: too hot, too cold, too rainy. It might be a work project that needs just a little more time. A headache. A phone call from a child who wants a ride home. Dinner to prepare. You wonder if it's worth it to squeeze in a walk.

A choice to follow the "high road" delivers an even steeper challenge when the decision is muddied by addictions. It's a turning point confronted every evening by a Virginia wife and mother whose relaxing glass of wine after work has fed a dependency. "I would like to consider myself a problem drinker, but according to Alcoholics Anonymous, I'm an alcoholic," says the woman I'll call Suzanne. "I've abused alcohol for many years, and that doesn't work well with the motivation to walk. I'm able to drink or not drink, but once I take a drink, I drink way too much. There seems to be a shut-off switch missing."

The "switch" Suzanne needed came when she said yes to an invitation to participate in a long-distance walk to benefit breast cancer. She agreed to join a sister-in-law who had recently completed breast cancer treatment. With a team of family walkers, Suzanne began training to walk thirty-nine miles in two days as a participant in New York City's Avon Walk for Breast Cancer. It quickly became clear that she wouldn't make it out of the house for training walks if she lifted a wineglass first. Instead of reaching for a glass as soon as she got home from work, Suzanne put on her walking shoes. Walking to benefit a worthy cause did more than change the rhythm of a daily habit. Within four months, the exercise and a wine-free diet also brought personal benefits of weight loss and energy gain, she says.

When the two-day walk was over, she faced the end of a workday with new resolve. The solutions weren't simple, but walking had sharpened awareness of the choices she could make. Now, she says, participation in AA meetings and regular walks help her maintain balance in the daily struggle to take the "high road" with alcohol. "I must admit, there are still days when I vacillate," she concedes. "At the end of the day, is it wine or walk? That's the question. I can't have both." On those days Suzanne shuts out temptation with earphones, letting music reinforce a willful effort to take the high road.

Whether you put on a headset or tune your own mind to the task of making up lyrics as I often do, music can be a powerful ally when willpower wavers. It can deliver momentum that carries you past the temptation of a glass of wine, the lure of a new magazine, or the enticing pull of inertia. Combine the cadence of your steps with the rhythms of a song, and you strengthen the harmonizing flow of energy that restores wholeness for body and spirit.

Sidewalk Songwriting

On this walking program, you've been urged to make time for silence in your daily walks. Silence allows you to integrate mind and body in the healing steps you are taking—to hear the wisdom of your spirit or your conscience. When healing or integration is a goal on your walks, silence supports you. It creates a space in which to reconnect with yourself. Often the first form of healing we need in hard times is the recovery of wholeness, healing the fragmentation that trauma delivers.

But there's a time and a place for music, too—especially music you make in your own head. Research demonstrates that music encourages exercisers to work out harder and longer. So take advantage of that assistance when you need some extra support to overcome a slump in energy or willpower. Before you put on a headset and leave the musical creativity to someone else, why not become a sidewalk composer?

On the Walking Well program, you've already experimented with walks that establish a three-count pattern for steps and breath. If you're a waltz lover, you might have found yourself humming along mentally with your count. My standard waltz tune is Strauss's "Blue Danube Waltz," which I play over and over in my head as I walk, counting *In-two-tree, Out-two-three*, while the melody gently lifts my energy. Sometimes the count shifts into the words of personalized lyrics I create for the well-known waltz. *I am here, I am strong, Yes, I am, Yes, I am,* I sing to myself. *I am here, Mov-ing on, Yes, I am, Yes, I am.* The "Blue Danube" flows smoothly through my cells, flooding me with air and optimism. On days when the path is smooth, the feel-good chemicals wash over me and I glide on the notes of my own three-beat Endorphin Waltz: *En-dor-phins, en-dor-phins, in my blood, feel so good; en-dor-phins, en-dor-phins, give me more, let me soar.*

The words pull my thoughts away from chores and errands and to-do lists. They block the worries that feed anxiety. For a few minutes, I am present and lifted, both physically and emotionally, on the rhythms of a song. It's playful and it's healing. But keep the singing inside your head. Singing or talking aloud as you walk disrupts a regular pattern of full, steady breathing. You're likely to wind up out of breath or hunched over with a side-ache.

Songwriting is cognitive override you can personalize. Change the words to suit your mood. Change the tune when you change terrain.

Songwriting offers a form of cognitive override that you can personalize as often as you want. Change the words to suit your state of mind or the conditions of the day. Change your tune when you change terrain. Heading up a steep street or hillside, you may find it helpful to match your steps and your breath to a slow, steady rhythm. I stumbled upon the motivational side of a children's song one day after visiting a friend whose young daughter had just received a new toy—a mechanical music box that pumped out "Old MacDonald" while barnyard animals circled the dial. The childhood tune returned to my thoughts as I plodded up the last two blocks of a steep pitch on my neighborhood walking route. As usual, the climb launched mental protests. *Ugh, this is hard. My legs are heavy.* Then something shifted. "Old MacDonald" rolled into my head, triggering new lyrics for this occasion. *One step for-ward at a time, one step up I climb,* I sang mentally. A simple ditty had the power to block the protests in my brain, and lead me home with a light heart.

When events in life push the stress levels up, music delivers more than motivation. Music can contribute a healing release. Participants in an Italian research project lowered blood pressure and stress levels by listening to music thirty minutes a day while matching breathing patterns to the music. Researchers concluded that full, rhythmic breathing produced the reduction in blood pressure readings, and they credit music with providing a tool to guide a regular breathing pattern.[3] Probably something much the same happened when I let "Old MacDonald" take my mind off the stress of self-criticism on my hike. With the rhythm of the children's song to steady my breathing, oxygen levels went up, and stress went down.

When stress goes down, you may encounter a lighter spirit inside. A few years ago, I was walking a trail flanked with towering evergreens as I prepared for a walking workshop in the Big Sky area of Montana. Rays of sunlight streamed through breaks in the trees, splashing the trail with fingers of light. It was a good day to be alive. A great day to be outdoors. As I walked, I heard the notes of "Zippity Do Dah" circling in my brain. Soon I had my own words for the tune playing in my head: *Puttin' my foot down, gatherin' pep. Movin' forward and takin' a step.* OK—it's not Grammy material, but it was fun. It was a way to integrate my mood, and my intention, into a rhythm that energized me.

Sometimes you may decide you need more help than you can muster by yourself. On those occasions, you may choose to rely on a portable music player. That's OK. The first priority is to make walking a regular, reliable pattern in your life. Anything that gets you moving will support your well-being and healing. Use the tools you need, but use them wisely. Music players lend energy when your goal is a walking workout. I plug into music on days when my primary goal is to maintain an aerobic pace.

But when my goal on a walk is peace of mind, or clarity, the music has to come from within. It's a matter of using the tool that's most appropriate for the outcome you seek.

For times when recorded music is your choice, put together a collection of instrumental music. Because the rhythmic pattern of walking encourages stress release, a musical beat can help you set and maintain a consistent tempo. Select melodies without lyrics so that you can fit your own affirmative phrases and positive self-talk to the beat of the song. Mentally, create personalized lyrics that motivate you or support your health, your strength, your safety, or your goals. No judgment! Just allow the rhythm and your own creativity to guide you. For safety, use music players only in areas where you feel secure, and always keep one ear free so that you remain aware of traffic or other activity around you.

Chants, prayers, and mantras are also rhythm makers. Buddhist pilgrims who recite "Om mani padme hum" as they circle holy sites experience a rhythmic repetition of words and steps that calms the mind. Repetitions of the rosary produce the same effect. Often a kind of singsong melody emerges from the repetition of a prayer so that the words rise and fall in a musical sequence that adds another level to the pattern.

Perhaps you will want to listen, in the silence of a walk, for an uplifting phrase that can echo the rhythm of your breath and steps. *Ho-ly Spir-it, Come-to-me* shaped a meaningful cadence for a participant in one of my walking seminars. *Give me wis-dom, give me pa-tience* is a four-beat prayer I lean on when I'm feeling uncertain or restless. The words calm the prickly tempo of fear that spurs anxiety, and bring a soothing focus to my thoughts.

Where we place our thoughts determines what we become.

Where we place our thoughts determines what we become, the Buddha advised his followers 2,000 years ago.[4] As he thinketh in his heart, so is he, the Bible concurs.[5] Science confirms that thoughts impact body chemistry. Biofeedback monitors reveal changes in blood pressure when thoughts switch from anxious to placid. Music engages both the brain and the motor system, smoothing out movements of people who have motor disorders like Parkinson's disease. Perhaps, simply by directing thoughts away from worries and fears and turning them to words of inspiration or spiritual guidance, we shift the course of our own healing. Combine those words with music, and healing pulses through every cell.

SIDE STEPS: *Walking and Joints*

Not all of the body's 143 joints get activated when you take a walk, but plenty of them are involved. From the neck to the shoulder and down to the toes, we rely on joints for the mobility that lets us take steps. But it's a mutual relationship—the body's moving parts rely on us just as much as we rely on them. Movement keeps them in working order.

Movement triggers production of synovial fluid, the lubricant that is essential to smooth joint function. Increased circulation of blood and lymph in the joints supplies nutrients that clean and heal tissues. Sprains and strains may interfere with exercise from time to time, but even these injuries respond favorably to moderate exercise as the healing begins. A more persistent and pervasive joint complaint results from osteoarthritis—a chronic condition caused by inflammation and loss of cartilage in the joints. The Centers for Disease Control reports that one in five Americans has been diagnosed with osteoarthritis. In many cases, osteoarthritis is caused by wear and tear on the joints, which means it tends to show up as people age.

Many medical experts claim that exercise provides some protection against the development of osteoarthritis by helping to reduce body weight, strengthening shock-absorbing muscles and ligaments around joints, and increasing flexibility. Research soundly supports exercise as a means of managing the pain of arthritis for those who have already developed symptoms. The Johns Hopkins Arthritis Center stresses that "physical activity is essential to optimizing both physical and mental health and can play a vital role in the management of arthritis."[6]

Posture and a few corrective exercises can help you minimize stress on your joints as you walk.

POSTURE

Take care to hold your body upright, spine and neck reaching toward the sky. Keeping the upper body erect helps maintain good alignment of joints in the lower body as you walk. Pretend you are zipping up the front of your slacks to pull your tummy in. That movement helps tuck the buttocks into a position that supports your lower back.

STRIDE

Short steps reduce impact on your knee joints. When you keep the stride length short, you can focus on using your foot as a roller to cushion each step. Keep your body movement forward, with hips level rather than dropping from side to side with each step.

KNEE JOINT

For strength and stability in the knee joint, both the quadriceps muscles in the front of the thigh and the hamstring muscles on the back of the thigh must be strong and balanced. If either side is weak, knee stability is compromised. By strengthening these muscles, you protect the knee. This is a step you can take sitting down. Choose a straight-backed chair and sit with both feet flat on the floor. Lift one leg straight out in front of you, as high as you can. Bend the knee and lower the foot back to the floor. Lift again and straighten the leg, this time turning the sole of your foot in toward the center of your body. Lower the foot, and lift a final time, turning the sole of your foot out, away from the midline. Build up to do the lifts ten times on each leg.

When walking on steep downhill slopes, keep your knees bent so thigh muscles absorb impact, and zigzag on the trail to reduce direct, downhill pressure on the knees.

ANKLE JOINT

To strengthen muscles that support the ankle, begin with simple rotations of the foot. Sitting on a straight chair, raise the foot and circle the toes several times in both directions. Repeat with the opposite foot. These easy circles help lubricate the ankle joint and increase flexibility.

At the end of a walk, when muscles are warmed up, take the opportunity to strengthen your ankles by standing on a step with a banister—perhaps at your front door. Position the balls of your feet side by side on the step and hold the rail for balance. Your heels will hang over the edge of the step. Lower your heels and then lift up onto the balls of the feet. Build up to ten times.

Dancers need music, but walkers are their own music.

—W. A. Mathieu, *The Listening Book*

When you walk, your footsteps create a rhythm you can hear and feel. Scuff a toe and the rhythm changes. On a hill, the rhythm slows. At the corner, it rests as you wait for the traffic to pass. Pick up the pace and you find a new rhythm. Behind it all lies the beat of your heart, a steady drummer for the rhythms of life. Walking is always a rhythmic exercise, but this week, you'll bring some variety to the tempo of your steps. You'll be waltzing and marching as you accompany your steps with mental music that sustains the beat. Whether counting, singing, or writing your personal lyrics, you set your cells in motion.

Rhythm operates as a fundamental monitor of our most primary body functions. It emerges in breathing patterns, pulse, heart rate, stress response, and sleep cycles, as well as in walking styles. There is reassurance in rhythm. A pattern of repetition offers continuity and safety—a cycle we can rely on. When life events disrupt those rhythms, we may experience fear, anger, confusion, or grief. That's when it can be helpful to return to the rhythms that remain constant in our lives. Walking calms emotional unrest by restoring connection with the rhythm of your steps, your heart, your breath.

Mark Liponis, MD, Medical Director for Canyon Ranch health resorts, recommends that all of us have some form of rhythmic exercise five times a week. "It reduces stress, increases stamina, relaxes the body and mind, slows the aging process, and improves the health of the immune system," he says.[7] When you add music, exercise becomes even more rhythmic, Liponis says. "You will notice more spring in your step. You will swing your arms differently. Exercise will take less effort. And you feel you have more stamina. Add to that that you are no longer worrying about things undone or things to come. And it's fun."

As you practice putting some rhythmic variety in your walks

this week, you'll be exercising both brain and body. The four-beat pattern is most common in music we hum automatically. When you vary your walking rhythm by inserting a three-count sometimes, the lead shifts from side to side. Left and right feet alternate the lead in the rhythm of 1-2-3. Because sides of the body correlate with sides of the brain, a three-count pace also balances activity in the brain.

1. WALTZ WALKING

You've been experimenting with a three-beat walking cadence for a few weeks, and by now the rhythm is probably comfortable. This week, see if you can expand the three-beat walk by adding a mental melody to accompany your count. If you know a few bars of Strauss's "Blue Danube Waltz," try playing the melody in your head to set the pattern of your steps. Or use the opening measures of "My Favorite Things" for a different three-count rhythm. "Greensleeves" offers another option. And then there's the holiday sing-along "Over the River and Through the Woods." Let yourself play a bit with this three-beat experiment. Vary the tempo. Slow it down or speed it up to make it a smooth metronome for your steps. You may discover that some of your own favorite songs provide the same soothing beat.

2. FOUR-STEP CADENCE, SOUSA STYLE

If you played an instrument in your high school marching band, you'll have no problem coming up with a suitable four-beat melody to set the pace for this exercise. "Stars and Stripes" is a familiar march, but many other tunes work just as well. The four-beat is a common rhythm for much of the music we know.

"Yankee Doodle" is a British folk song that has become an American standard. It's an easy starting place for a four-beat pairing of music and movement. Once you get the melody in mind, accentuate the count by repeating *In-two-three-four, Out-two-three-four* mentally. When you say the numbers, you create a mindful cadence of melody, breath, and steps that deepens stress release.

But if you can't get the words out of your head, don't give up. You are blocking words of worry and fear with lyrics that block out automatic stressors. Whenever your mind drifts away to other thoughts, make a willful effort to pull yourself back to the rhythm. You'll increase relaxation and stress release by closing your mind to self-doubt and criticism.

Other familiar four-beat songs you might try include "It's a Grand Old Flag" or "The Girl from Ipanema." If you're not in the mood for a lighthearted tune, find a song that comforts you. Perhaps you'll find stability in the rhythms of a favorite hymn. Match the rhythmic cadence of the Beatles with "All You Need Is Love" or "Let It Be." Or let "Every Time I Feel the Spirit" lift your mood and energy.

3. EVERY LITTLE CELL

You may be familiar with this four-beat variation on the folk song "Shortnin' Bread." It's been circling through support groups, church circles, and youth camps. In this case, both words and rhythm lead you on a healing journey. Lots of variations exist, so change the words to suit yourself. Remember to keep the song in your head, and to keep your breathing regular. You may not get a clear cadence with this syncopated four-beat melody, and that's fine. Enjoy the energy of the song. Here's a version I like:

> Every little cell in my body is happy
> Every little cell in my body is well.
> Feels so good, feels so swell,
> Every little cell is well, well, well.

Previous Exercises You'll Use This Week

1. BREATHE IN, BREATHE OUT (WEEK ONE)

Mentally remind yourself *In* as you inhale and *Out* as you exhale. Focusing awareness on the words and breath speeds the release of stress.

2. THREE-STEP: IN-2-3 CADENCE (WEEK THREE)

Mentally, repeat *In-two-three, Out-two-three* to establish a three-beat cadence of breath, steps, and words. If you start on the right foot with *In-two-three,* then the left foot takes the lead on *Out-two-three.* Stay focused to avoid drifting into the more familiar four-count with *In-two-three*-pause, *Out-two-three*-pause.

3. FOUR-STEP: IN-2-3-4 CADENCE (WEEK TWO)

Keep your walks interesting and your rhythm varied by returning to the four-count cadence: *In-two-three-four, Out-two-three-four.*

4. SAY THANK YOU (WEEK ONE)

Choose the rhythm of gratitude as you end each walk with appreciation. Gratitude becomes a four-beat chant by pairing steps with a four-syllable phrase: *I am grate-ful.* For a three-beat cadence, try *I give thanks.* Let yourself feel appreciation for things that support and enrich your life today. Caring friends, good books, a loyal pet, a loving spouse, a warm home. Appreciation, like oxygen, is an antidote to stress. Use it often.

Week Five Goals Overview

Walk Level	Walk Time Goal	Silent Segment Time Goal
Stepping Out	Walk 6 days 15–18 min. a day	10 min. silent
Mid-Stride	Walk 6 days 25 min. 4 days 20 min. 2 days	15–20 min. silent
Strong and Steady	Walk 6 days 30 min. 4–5 days 40 min. 1–2 days	20–30 min. silent

Week Five Daily Walk Guidelines

Rotate walks at your level for variety during the week. Try walks at a different level if you want more or less exercise. You are always welcome to extend walks if you are feeling stronger. Add a previous technique that you have enjoyed, or extend the suggested timing for these focus tools.

Stepping Out		
Week 5	Focusing Techniques Rotate routines for variety	Suggested Timing
2 days 15–18 min.	1. Breathe In, Breathe Out 2. Three-Step: In-2-3 Cadence 3. Waltz Walking: In-2-3 Cadence 4. Say Thank You	5 min. 5 min. 6 min. 2 min.
2 days 15–18 min.	1. Three-Step: In-2-3 Cadence 2. Four-Beat Cadence, Sousa Style 3. Every Little Cell 4. Say Thank You	5 min. 5 min. 5 min. 3 min.
2 days 15–18 min.	1. Three-Step: In-2-3 Cadence 2. Four-Step: In-2-3-4 Cadence 3. Waltz Walking: In-2-3 Cadence 4. Say Thank You	5 min. 5 min. 5 min. 3 min.

Mid-Stride		
Week 5	Focusing Techniques Rotate routines for variety	Suggested Timing
4 days 25 min.	1. Breathe In, Breathe Out Or: Walk, Talk, Listen 2. Three-Step: In-2-3 Cadence 3. Waltz Walking: In-2-3 Cadence 4. Every Little Cell 5. Say Thank You	5 min. 10 min. 8 min. 2 min.
2 days 20 min.	1. Four-Step: In-2-3-4 Cadence 2. Four-Beat Cadence, Sousa Style 3. Every Little Cell 4. Say Thank You	6 min. 6 min. 6 min. 2 min.

Strong and Steady		
Week 5	Focusing Techniques Rotate routines for variety	Suggested Timing
4–5 days 30 min.	1. Breathe In, Breathe Out Or: Walk, Talk, Listen 2. Three-Step: In-2-3 Cadence 3. Waltz Walking: In-2-3 Cadence 4. Four-Step: In-2-3-4 Cadence 5. Say Thank You	10 min. 6 min. 6 min. 6 min. 2 min.
1–2 days 40 min.	1. Four-Step: In-2-3-4 Cadence Or: Walk, Talk, Listen 2. Four-Beat Cadence, Sousa Style 3. Every Little Cell 4. Three-Step: In-2-3 Cadence 5. Waltz Walking: In-2-3 Cadence 6. Say Thank You	10 min. 7 min. 7 min. 7 min. 7 min. 2 min.

Log In

Make a daily note on the Week Five log about your walking time, your mood, and your thoughts or observations after each walk. Keeping a log encourages you to walk with awareness.

- How did it feel to waltz walk this week? Does music help you sustain a three-count cadence? What song did you find most helpful?
- Which did you find easier, the waltz cadence or the march?
- What do you feel grateful for today?
- Does the rhythm of music affect your mood in any way?
- What did you learn about yourself on this walk?
- Did you create a personal song?

Week Six

A Healthy Attitude

> Trauma is a demanding tutor, urging us to learn fresh ways to look at life. It prompts us to ask new questions: What gives my life purpose now? Where do I find meaning? This week, make a choice to move forward toward a new point of view. Your steps launch a shift of position that reverberates in attitude.

*F*or Carolee Shaw, trauma came in the form of an automobile accident—the consequences of one driver more focused on a cell phone conversation than on the stop sign ahead. The collision hurled Carolee's car into a telephone pole and changed forever the trajectory of her life.

A college professor with a doctorate in speech communication, she had relied on sharp mental skills for both professional success and personal satisfaction. She breezed through a couple of novels a week for relaxation and designed innovative courses for students at the University of Colorado in Denver.

In the instant of impact, all that changed. She emerged from the accident unable to make sense of the words in a newspaper. Unable to figure out the messages delivered by a television newscaster. At first the confusion was hard to explain. The accident had produced no visible injuries, and a cursory hospital examination did not reveal the traumatic brain damage in both the frontal and parietal lobes that future tests disclosed. Twelve years after the accident, she acknowledges that the damage is permanent.

"Now I work as a file clerk at the Museum of Science and Nature in Denver," she says.[1] "The injury has been very humbling. To learn something new is painful. Sometimes I give up trying to learn and say, 'I think I know enough to get me through the rest of my life.' It's just too hard to learn now."

Because she can no longer learn by reading—the jumble of words on a printed page simply does not produce meaningful sentences or thoughts for her anymore—Carolee has found new ways to learn. Walking revealed a path of learning; nature has been her classroom.

"Walking helps," she says. "It forces me to get out of the house and feel the air and feel that I am alive. When I walk, I make myself very aware of what is around me and how it feels. If it's windy, I am aware of the wind on my face, in my hair, or moving in the leaves. It's a new source of information about the world around me."

By focusing outward—on the wind, the birds, a brilliant flower—Carolee pushed past the doubts and depression that haunted her in the wake of a chance encounter with an inattentive driver. Instead of clinging to regrets about the loss of mental clarity, professional status, relationships, and self-image, she turned her attention to the world outside herself. The walks gave structure to days left shapeless by the loss of a university position and the distancing of friends unable to connect with the new person Carolee had become.

"Walking has been very helpful to me because I use it as a daily goal," she says. "I use it for stimulation. What I did was, I became more a part of nature, and that helped me realize that I belonged in the world. Also, I became aware of what I have control over and what I don't have control over. I do have control over my awareness. I can choose to go out and walk around the block and ignore everything outside myself, or I can choose to become aware of what's around me. Nature has become my learning tool."

As she traveled the sidewalks of her Denver neighborhood, Carolee began noticing the distinct calls of different birds. She learned to recognize the whistle of a chickadee and the song of a mourning dove. Cautiously, she began to offer a response as she walked her daily route. She mimicked the birds she heard most often and practiced until her message produced replies from the birds she encountered on her path.

"It was thrilling," she says. "It became fun—a form of communication, that made walking even more delightful."

Choose to Make a Choice

By walking, Carolee began to reclaim control in one small corner of her life. Her decision to walk contributed to both physical and emotional recovery. Choice, large or small, constitutes a cornerstone of resiliency. Every choice strengthens the awareness that some things remain within one's sphere of control. Every choice affirms a way in which you still can make a difference in your life and in your world.

"Choice is the father of freedom, and the voice of the heart," maintains psychologist Dan Baker, author of *What Happy People Know*.[2] Baker suffered his own collision with tragedy at the death of his infant son. The experience guided a personal and professional focus on the tools of resiliency that he shares in his book and in his work as a therapist. "Having no choices, or options, feels like being in jail," he says.

Choice, large or small, constitutes a cornerstone of resiliency.

It's true, many options are taken away by a serious illness or a disaster. We feel boxed in, confined, and limited by conditions we can't control. But some choices remain. Even inside the confines of a physical jail, we see examples of people who manage to find choice. Some choose to pursue an education. Some become bodybuilders. Some, like celebrity homemaker Martha Stewart, share their skills behind bars. When sentenced to five months in federal prison for lying about an investment scheme, Stewart taught fellow inmates to knit. She found a way to take control in one small corner of her life and in doing so, maintained a sense of purpose. The challenge is to see those opportunities for choice and to take action. Any action. A decision to act begins to lift the weight of helplessness that often accompanies a trauma.

"Everything can be taken from a man but one thing: the last of the human freedoms—to choose one's attitude in any given set of circumstances, to choose one's own way," writes Holocaust survivor Viktor Frankl.[3] Confined three years in Nazi concentration camps, Frankl observed that prisoners who had a sense of purpose or intention were more likely to survive the horrors of the camps. Whether purpose came through love for another person, a work role, or a spiritual belief, it gave a person something to live for . . . it gave life meaning when the world seemed bleak and hopeless. An Austrian neurologist and psychiatrist, Frankl emerged from the camps in 1945 with a passionate belief in the importance of personal choice.

With his book *Man's Search for Meaning*, Frankl has inspired readers around the world who feel caught in the prison of illness, depression, pain, or grief. "We must never forget that we may also find meaning in life even when confronted with a hopeless situation, when facing a fate that cannot be changed," he wrote. "When we are no longer able to change a situation—think of an incurable disease such as inoperable cancer—we are challenged to change ourselves."[4]

For Carolee Shaw, change began with a decision to step back into the world with walks through her neighborhood. When faced with brain damage she could not reverse, she turned attention outward, to the natural world around her. The change launched a shift in attitude that helped her redefine her life. Gradually, it expanded a world that seemed tragically narrowed by her accident.

"I'm definitely not the same person I was, but that's OK. It really seems that when one door appears to close, your values change, if you let it happen, and you gain new awareness," she says. "For me, the key, I think, has been to listen—to listen at a level that I didn't listen before. To listen to what's going on around me and to remember to be grateful, because I still have a lot to be grateful for."

New awareness isn't always easy, she admits. It has brought her to a firsthand understanding of how the world treats people in different work roles. People who once would have made a point of saying hello to her in respect for her education and university teaching position now breeze past her without a glance, not considering that an office clerk might have a doctorate degree.

"I used to know how the people at the top felt. Now I know how the janitors feel. It's interesting how we treat one another, without even realizing it. If this had not happened to me, I would have ended up being an intellectual snob. Now I don't judge people like I used to," she says.

Toward a New Point of View

New awareness, or new attitudes, aren't high on the priority list when crisis first hits. What we want in the upheaval of a traumatic event is for things to return to "normal." To go back to the patterns and behaviors and relationships we have known, even if they have been difficult.

"Often I see that people in trauma are frozen," says psychologist Baker. "I would encourage people who are traumatized to get up and get moving. Because of brain chemistry, movement produces a different response in the body than if you are sitting in a chair. So let's get them fluid. Let's get them moving, literally."[5]

When Baker works with people in crisis, he often sends them out into the world with an assignment to look around and identify half a dozen things or experiences they consider beautiful. Write them down, he says, making notes about why this item or activity is attractive.

"We have to go consciously, to look for the little miracles around us," he says. "There are little miracles to be found every day, whether in a smile, a loving comment, or the ripple of light on a stream." A walker who focuses on what can be seen, heard, or felt is making a continuous string of choices. The information coming to you through the eyes, ears, nose, and skin provides a form of meditative focus that temporarily blocks out worry and fear.

Never ask, "Why me?" Ask, "What can I learn from this?"

"We need to be aware that when one is traumatized, there is a pull into oneself, into the black hole," says psychologist Baker. "Even though it doesn't feel good, the pull is there. The moment you put your focus on something or someone else, it lifts you out of that. I don't think that people ever completely get past a trauma. The issue is that happy people pay the tuition. They ask 'what can I learn from my trauma?'"

Never ask "why me?" Baker stresses. There is no constructive answer to that question. In fact, the very question helps keep you stuck in the trauma rather than moving through it. Instead, ask:

- What do I need right now?
- What are my resources?
- What can I do to become more resilient?
- What can I learn from this?

Then find a way to shift your focus, even briefly, away from your questions and fears. Take a walk and focus intently on the miracles of life outside you, in the way that Carolee did. The physical steps of a walk help break the imprisonment of fear and grief. They help you find a reason to go on.

Walking Toward the Light

Several years ago, I made a leap of faith and signed up for a twenty-eight-day trek in Nepal. Physical challenges were new to me at that point in my life. Hiking appealed to the fresh, new athlete awakening in me—exotic travel combined with a spiritual quest. The itinerary promised three weeks of trekking, from a village in the Himalayan foothills to the glaciers of Everest Base Camp. Along the way, we would visit monasteries in remote villages untouched by roadways and camp in tent villages set up by sherpas. I envisioned inspiring encounters with spiritual masters. But it was an American guide who taught me the most about an enlightened attitude.

A combination motivational leader and athletic coach, Linda Williamson was one of three leaders on the Nepal trek. She brought to the task both physical and mental strength—the result of years spent exploring the challenges of nature, whether guiding whitewater rafting trips or inviting hikers to investigate physical and spiritual heights. Her ease with the discomforts of camping and aching ascents alerted the skeptic in me initially. But before the trek reached its culmination, I had come to value Linda's skills. From her I learned how to push beyond the discomfort and self-doubt of an outdoors beginner. How to use my head to help support my body. How to let a song take my focus off the steep pitch ahead when my spirit faltered and my steps began to plod.

Now Linda is the one who plods—each step possible only with support from the braces that wrap her legs. For two years, she has been losing her physical strength to the advances of amyotrophic lateral sclerosis (ALS), also called Lou Gehrig's disease. ALS is a degenerative disease that affects nerve cells, gradually destroying the ability of the brain to communicate with muscle fibers. Early symptoms often include muscle weakness. Linda's ALS symptoms began with muscles in the neck and throat, an unusual form of the disease. Slurred speech was a first indication of something gone awry.

Ten days after her diagnosis of ALS, she and her husband strapped on rollerblades and skated ninety miles across Idaho.

They had been training for the distance event and used it as a route through the immobilizing shock of a medical crisis. For five days of skating, the steady rhythm of their movement carried them through the fog of uncertainty and grief.

"Given that rollerblading has been one of my passions in life, I found that skating in a beautiful, serene environment really helped my emotional state," she says.[6] "I was in total bliss some of the time, not living in devastation. Ralph and I loved being together, sharing this experience. I believe that because of the skating, and the diagnosis, we fell more in love with each other and ourselves."

Like walking, skating produces repetitive, rhythmic movement that encourages stress release in the body. It boosts oxygen intake, heart rate, and circulation, renewing essential resources. But Linda skated for more than exercise. "The long, slow glide of skating is the most freeing sense of being I have ever had," she says. "I always felt like I was dancing when I was skating."

As the disease progressed, muscles in the rest of her body have been affected. Two years after her diagnosis, she can no longer rollerblade. No longer talk, swallow food, or breathe on her own at night. She communicates with e-mail and an electronic voice machine, and with the light that still brightens her eyes. The gradual erosion of physical strength reveals the progression of her disease, moving slowly down the body from throat to toes. With no known cure for this illness, the course of ALS is inevitable.

When options have been explored, medications tested, experts consulted, prayers lofted upward around the world by chains of loving friends, there comes an awareness that all we can control is the present moment. Possibilities turn to finding meaning on the path that remains. Healing takes a different direction.

Even as Linda feels her body retreating, she holds fiercely to life by turning her focus to her breath, the very essence of spirit and being. And, when she is able, she continues to seek the healing that comes with walking. Supported by leg braces and the firm arm of her husband, she musters the strength for brief excursions into the world around her. The steps reconnect her with an image of herself as capable and comfortable in her body.

"I feel as if I am still normal when I am out walking," she says, explaining in an e-mail interview why she refuses to give up. "I seek to know that I can still move, explore, notice, and give gratitude for all the beauty of life outside. I believe the greatest gift of a walk is the actual breathing in, which is inhaling the divine air of life. And then breathing back out, honoring the circle of life."

She draws inner strength from the environment that challenged, inspired, taught, and nurtured her during her days as an outdoor guide. The creativity and spirit that once led her up Himalayan inclines now mold her approach to each day. "Being outside in nature is what keeps me doing our walks," she says. "What I love the most about nature is the light. Everywhere I look, even on darker days, there is light reflecting something positive someplace. I just need to look around. As I walk, my rhythmic movement is returned as I seek to follow the light."

Psychologists identify people like Linda as "hardy," meaning they find ways to overcome despair. Even when they can't control the situation, can't wait for a cure, they take control of attitude and of the choices they can make. Characteristics of hardy people include:

- Ability to see challenge in a situation rather than insurmountable threat.
- Ability to control attitude when unable to control circumstances.
- Ability to find commitment and purpose in life—a reason to move ahead.

In a symbolic way, all difficulties encourage us to look for the light—to look for what has the power to lead us out of darkness.

It doesn't take a devastating disease like ALS to call forth the need for hardiness. After the initial shock and numbness subside, periods of crisis force us to reevaluate. What really matters in our lives? Where do we want to place our focus? In a symbolic way, all difficulties encourage us to look for the light—to look around and see what still has the power to lead us out of darkness, out of fear, out of hopelessness. What light can chase the shadows from the path, even for a moment? What light gives purpose and reason to go on?

The "light" that Linda seeks on sidewalks, or leaves, or reflected from a windowpane is what we all need when we are plunged into a dark place in life. Looking for the light literally becomes a powerful focusing tool that opens the mind to the present moment. It is a form of meditation, or a tool of cognitive override. It is a means of temporarily silencing concerns and bringing focus to the vitality of nature, the essence of life that exists around us right now.

As Linda surrenders to the inexorable progression of her disease, she holds firmly to the life remaining. Her days will be filled with light, she insists. With laughter, and no tears. "I spend very little time wishing I was different now . . . or feeling sad because I can't do something," she says. "That seems like a waste of time because I can't change it, only accept it. Spiritually, I seem to be growing more aware of when I am fully present with what is than I used to be, because all I have is *right now* to enjoy."

Once again, as in Nepal, she points the way forward on an unfamiliar and difficult trek. She inspires my steps anew. I think of her and move ahead in search of light. I find it in the orange glow of a garden nasturtium, among the shadows that slide below the oak tree at the corner, in the shimmer of dew on a crisp morning. Light weaves a cord that leads me forward, in a game of hide and seek. It opens my eyes and brightens my spirit. It brings me present—an explorer on life's mysterious landscape, aware of *what is* right now. In those flashes of light, those moments of awareness, I am walking behind Linda, learning that when we can't change the path, we still can change our awareness of what remains. When the course of life is beyond our control, we make the choices that we can. A choice to focus on the light.

SIDE STEPS: *Walking and Brains*

Of course you know that exercise can increase the size of your muscles, but did you know that it can also help you grow a bigger brain? Or that it helps the brain you have work better? Walking even improves your ability to come up with facts and dates and people's names by enhancing memory skills. And it's never too late to start. Research shows that exercise can actually reverse brain shrinkage, healing the mental wear and tear that was once regarded as an inevitable side effect of life.

The mental benefits of walking result primarily from an enhanced flow of blood and oxygen. An increase in oxygen is almost always accompanied by a boost in mental sharpness. Circulation wakes up the brain cells, fuels them for action, and enables them to function more efficiently. Exercise also spurs the brain to produce a protein (brain-derived neurotropic factor) that encourages brain cells to grow, connect, and communicate.[7] Studies suggest that exercise even stimulates production of new brain cells, particularly in a part of the brain involved in learning and memory skills.

To stimulate creative problem solving and enhance clarity when you face important decisions, take a walk. Even five minutes at a brisk pace sharpens mental alertness. You'll come back better prepared to find solutions and make wise decisions.

BRAIN BUILDER

Walking spurs the growth of enough new nerve cells, or neurons, to produce a measurable increase in the size of people's brains in just six months, reports a study in the *British Journal of Sports Medicine*. Neurons are a core component of the brain and the spinal cord.[8] In this study, people who had been couch potatoes started with fifteen minutes of aerobic exercise, such as brisk walking, and built up to forty-five minutes, three times a week. "We found that walking will increase the volume of the brain, increase the efficiency of the brain, and increase improvements in a number of cognitive functions such as memory and attention," says researcher Arthur Kramer.[9]

MENTAL ALERTNESS

Researchers at the University of Illinois at Urbana-Champaign studied participants aged fifteen to seventy-one and confirmed that exercise brought improved mental activity, regardless of age. When participants were tested before and after an exercise program, researchers found that all ages showed faster response times and greater accuracy.[10] Authors of the study argue that results support the need for exercise in public schools and throughout adulthood.

REASONING AND DECISIONS

Clear thinking and the ability to make decisions improves for people who complete forty-five minutes of brisk walking three times a week. In a study funded by the National Council on Aging, participants aged sixty to seventy-five were tested on thinking skills before and after a six-month walking program. Walkers began with fifteen-minute walks three days a week and built up to forty-five-minute walks at a brisk pace, three days a week. Tests showed that walking program participants were mentally sharper in areas of planning, scheduling, and memory than participants in a control group who received stretching and toning exercise.[11]

REMEMBER THIS

Researchers in Australia found that walking for two and a half hours a week can significantly improve memory. Participants in a twenty-four-week trial of 170 people aged fifty and older were given instructions and educational materials on memory loss, stress management, and lifestyle factors that affect memory. Half of the group was instructed to walk for fifty minutes three times a week. The control group did not receive instructions to exercise. In tests at the end of the twenty-four-week period, walkers showed improvement in mental skills compared to the non-exercise group. The benefits continued for the walkers in tests administered one year after the trial.[12]

People usually consider walking on water or in thin air a
miracle. But I think the real miracle is not to walk
on water or in thin air, but to walk on earth.
Every day we are engaged in a miracle which we don't
even recognize: a blue sky, white clouds, green leaves,
the curious eyes of a child—our own two eyes.
All is a Miracle.

—Thich Nhat Hanh, *The Miracle of Mindfulness*

As we heal and begin to emerge from the tunnel vision of fear that trauma constructs, we often see life differently. Whether we see it with fresh appreciation or with resentment and resignation is a choice that we make. "We don't describe the world we see— we see the world we describe," says psychologist Dan Baker.[13] When it feels impossible to see the world differently, begin by moving your body, not your attitude. Movement triggers a chain of physical, mental, and emotional reactions that ease the passage to a larger perspective.

Buddhist monk Thich Nhat Hanh is a survivor of the Vietnam War. In the quote above, he views the world with the eyes of a survivor, reminding us that the miracle of life is all around us, if we can just see it. The message resonates with many survivors of trauma. Choose to look for the miracle this week with walks that lead you into nature in search of a new point of view.

Your senses are your body's gateway to the world around you. Sight, sound, smell, taste, touch—these are the tools that tell you where you are and what you are experiencing right now, in this moment. Carolee opened her senses to the song of birds and the natural beauty of a city park and found a path through grief and self-pity. Linda put her focus on light and followed its glow on leaves, and streams, and sidewalks as she traveled into the darkness of disease. Both found reassurance and purpose in their lives as they chose to focus on nature's bounty rather than on the restrictions that had restructured life for each of them.

1. SENSORY SCAN

Senses provide a very convenient means of staying mindful while moving. I use this process often to clear my head when I find my thoughts swirling during a walk. It is a method of getting present by paying attention to immediate surroundings, one sense at a time. Begin with a few full breaths, bringing air deep into the lungs and belly. Fresh air helps wake up the cells.

Now turn your focus to *vision*. Notice what you see as you walk. Maybe you become aware of cracks in the sidewalk. Perhaps it's a wildflower along the road. Be a mental reporter, sighting and taking note of what you see as you move along your route. Notice, too, that the sight of a dandelion can quickly trigger a gardening to-do list. When your thoughts lead you out of the moment, stop the intrusion with a gentle reminder—*Not now. Right now, I am here. I am seeing.* Try to hold your focus on what you see for a full minute, or perhaps for one block.

Then, shift awareness to your sense of *hearing*. Spend a few minutes or a block with attention fully attuned to the sounds around you. Make mental notes of the wind in the leaves overhead. Distant traffic on the freeway. The chatter of birds. The clinking of a dog's leash. Stay focused on sounds.

Next, switch to what you *smell* as you walk. Take big breaths, through the nose, to draw in air and aromas. If the fragrance of morning coffee from a neighbor's kitchen evokes memories of someone you miss, tell your mind, *Not now. Right now, I am here. I am smelling.* Move forward to pick up the next scent.

Finally, turn attention to what you *feel*. Notice the texture of the earth or pavement beneath your feet. Be aware of the warmth of the sun or the chill of the breeze. Can you feel the pull of shoelaces across the top of your foot? Does your jacket collar brush against your neck? Do you notice the muscles in your shins or tension in your shoulders? Just be aware.

This exercise lets you practice staying present, in your senses, minute by minute. It doesn't matter what order you use in scanning the senses. Just give each sense a fair share of your attention. By opening your sensory antennae as you walk, you pull your focus away from worries and stressors inside your head. As you focus on sight, sound, smell, and feeling, you become more aware and attentive to your body and your surroundings. Little by little, you expand your world, and your perspective. Give yourself several minutes for this exercise to allow time to experience each sense fully.

2. FOUR-COUNT SENSORY SCAN

This exercise is a variation on the sensory scan that uses the rhythmic cadence of steps and words to guide awareness. Try it to see if you find it helpful to use mental prompts. I like to use this version when my thoughts are too active to settle down without a reminder. Create the four-count cadence of *In-two-three-four, Out-two-three-four* to set your pace and breathing pattern. Then, use four-count phrases to hold attention and cadence. By saying I am here with each repetition, you remind yourself to stay present. Focus on each sense for two or three minutes, repeating the phrase:

> I am here and, I am see-ing.
>> (Four steps inhale, four steps exhale)
> I am here and, I am hear-ing.
> I am here and, I am feel-ing.
> I am here and, I am smell-ing.

3. GUIDING LIGHT

Follow the light as you walk, seeking evidence of the radiance that illuminates life and brightens attitudes, as Linda Williamson describes: "Everywhere I look, even on darker days, there is light reflecting something positive someplace. I just need to look around." Spend four or five minutes looking around as you walk. Let light be your guide, so your eye finds the flash of light that reflects from a puddle, or the glow that illuminates a leaf. Spend several minutes following the light, giving thanks for this evidence of life.

Previous Exercises You'll Use This Week

1. CLEAR THE AIR: FOUR-COUNT CADENCE (WEEK TWO)

Use the four-count cadence of *In-two-three-four, Out-two-three-four* to coordinate steps, breath, and mental focus. Replace the numbers with words: *Fresh air comes in. Stale air goes out.* Imagine that you are drawing in fresh energy, openness, and a willing attitude. Exhale the stale air and used-up ideas that you are ready to release. Let go of attitudes that no longer serve you.

2. MENTAL MARINADES: THREE- OR FOUR-COUNT CADENCE (WEEK THREE)

Pair your steps and your breath with a positive affirmation to flood your cells with a healing marinade.

For a three-count cadence, begin with *I am here, I am strong.*

For a four-count cadence, start with *I am here and, I am heal-ing.*

As you walk, maintain the cadence, but experiment with new words to find words that affirm your own state of mind. For example: *I am here, I am calm. I am here, I am safe.* Or try a four-count: *I am here and, I am hap-py.* Or *I am walk-ing, I am health-y.* Find your own marinade—a word or two that resonates with your goals and values.

3. SAY THANK YOU (WEEK ONE)

A moment of appreciation ends the walk with reminders of what is still working in your life. Maintain cadence with *I give thanks* (three-count) or *I am thank-ful* (four-count).

Week Six Goals Overview

Walk Level	Walk Time Goal	Silent Segment Time Goal
Stepping Out	Walk 6 days 16–20 min. a day	10 min. silent
Mid-Stride	Walk 6 days 25 min. a day	15–20 min. silent
Strong and Steady	Walk 6 days 30 min. 4–5 days 40 min. 1–2 days	20–30 min. silent

Week Six Daily Walk Guidelines

Rotate walks at your level for variety during the week. Use the suggested times as a starting place and make changes if you find a technique you want to practice longer, or if you want to alter the length of your walks. Experiment with all of the new techniques so that you keep adding new focusing skills to your cognitive override resources.

Stepping Out		
Week 6	Focusing Techniques Rotate routines for variety	Suggested Timing
2 days 16–20 min.	1. Sensory Scan 2. Mental Marinades 3. Say Thank You	10 min. 6–8 min. 2 min.
2 days 16–20 min.	1. Clear the Air: Four-Beat Cadence Or: Walk, Talk, Listen 2. Guiding Light 3. Say Thank You	10 min. 8 min. 2 min.
2 days 16–20 min.	1. Four-Count Sensory Scan 2. Mental Marinades 3. Say Thank You	10 min. 8 min. 2 min.

Mid-Stride		
Week 6	Focusing Techniques Rotate routines for variety	Suggested Timing
3 days 25 min.	1. Breathe In, Breath Out Or: Walk, Talk, Listen 2. Sensory Scan 3. Guiding Light 4. Say Thank You	5 min. 10 min. 8 min. 2 min.
3 days 25 min.	1. Clear the Air: Four-Beat Cadence Or: Walk, Talk, Listen 2. Four-Count Sensory Scan 3. Mental Marinades 4. Say Thank You	8 min. 10 min. 5 min. 2 min.

Strong and Steady		
Week 6	Focusing Techniques Rotate routines for variety	Suggested Timing
4–5 days 30 min.	1. Guiding Light Or: Walk, Talk, Listen 2. Sensory Scan 3. Mental Marinades 4. Say Thank You	8 min. 10 min. 10 min. 2 min.
1–2 days 40 min.	1. Breathe In, Breathe Out Or: Walk, Talk, Listen 2. Clear the Air: Four-Beat Cadence 3. Four-Count Sensory Scan 4. Guiding Light 5. Say Thank You	10 min. 10 min. 12 min. 6 min. 2 min.

Log In

Reinforce your daily discoveries by taking a minute or two to reflect on what made the walk significant. Record your thoughts and your walking time, on the walking log for Week Six.

- What did you discover about your environment as you explored it using the Sensory Scan exercise? What did you see, smell, or hear that made you smile?
- How did you feel when you started the walk? Did you feel better, worse, or unchanged at the end?
- How did it feel to let light be your guide on the route? What did you notice about light?
- What did you learn about yourself on this walk?
- What elicited gratitude?

By paying attention to these things, you begin to revitalize your relationship with yourself and with the world around you.

Week Seven

A Healthy Heart

Get to the heart of the matter this week with walks that touch your core, physically and emotionally. Strengthen your physical heart with a walking pace that builds cardiovascular health and enhances fitness. Open yourself to a change of heart with steps that lighten a heavy heart and warm a cold one.

*G*rowing up in a small western Kansas town, Elvira Valenzuela Crocker learned the value of exercise at an early age. In Garden City, softball offered more than vacant lot recreation— it provided a social environment where the child of a Mexican immigrant family could pitch her way to a position of respect.

As one of thirteen children, Elvira developed her throwing arm in backyard family games. From warm-up tosses for her brothers, she advanced to the mound of community softball teams before she turned her focus toward writing rather than athletics. Journalism carried her to Washington, D.C., where she held communications positions with the National Council of La Raza, the U.S. Commission on Civil Rights, the U.S. Department of Education, and the National Education Association. She served a term as national president of MANA, a Latina organization.

With family and career, her days were full and often long. Work-related travel fragmented her schedules and routines. Exercise slipped to a catch-as-catch-can status, and added pounds began padding her frame. Then a diagnosis of diabetes stopped her short. She knew the risks. "Hispanics have a high incidence of diabetes, as do blacks," she says. "As a diabetic, you always worry about heart problems, foot problems, kidney issues, and for me, eye issues. Because I am a writer and an avid reader, my biggest fear is the loss of my eyesight."[1]

Diabetes is the leading cause of blindness in people aged twenty to seventy-four, according to the American Diabetes Association. Diabetics are twice as likely to have heart disease as nondiabetics. Two out of three people with diabetes die from heart disease or stroke, the Diabetes Association reports.

Elvira's diagnosis dealt an emotional wallop in addition to frightening statistics. Two siblings—one brother and one sister—had already been diagnosed with diabetes by the time her condition was detected. Both have since died of heart disease. Her father, too, became diabetic late in life. Elvira responded to diabetes with the determination and sharp focus that had won her recognition both on the pitching mound and in the world of journalism.

"What I learned early on about diabetes is that it takes three things to manage it—diet, medication, and, importantly, exercise," she says. She took the message to heart, and now keeps blood sugar stable with a daily dose of all three. "I started by getting up early and walking on a school basketball court a block away from home before I went to work," she says. "What I found was that after a point, it didn't matter whether I felt like walking or not, my body just insisted on my daily fix of exercise. It demanded that I get out of bed at 6:30 AM to get my walk in."

With the daily walks and diet changes, she began to lose weight and gain strength. Before long, she expanded her walks. She added the four-block walk from home to the subway that took her to work in downtown Washington, D.C. When that was comfortable, she pushed herself to trek 1.8 miles from home to the next stop on the line at Chevy Chase before boarding the train.

"That solo walking prepared me for the day ahead," she says. "I could think through what I had to do and focus on my main writing assignment of the day. By the time I arrived at my desk, I was ready to hit the ground running." Weekday walks provided time for reflection and introspection. Weekends offered social contact as Elvira connected with neighbors for walks in the vicinity. She joined a fitness club and became a poster child for diabetic health. She shakes her head in disbelief at diabetics who rely on drugs and diet but omit exercise as a third tool for controlling blood sugar.

"Frankly, I just don't get it," she says. "Exercise makes me feel better. I find I have more energy when I exercise, my mood is fairly even, and it helps with weight control. Really, how hard is it? You pick up one foot and then the other. For me, exercise isn't optional. It's a matter of life and death."

Heart of the Matter

For years, medical advisors have publicized the link between exercise and heart disease. For years, physical activity guidelines from government sources have recommended aerobic activity to keep the heart in healthy working order. Yet heart disease is a leading cause of disability and death in the United States. Most of us don't pay much attention to the muscle that sustains our lives until something forces us to make changes in the way we live. It is estimated that 90 percent of coronary heart disease patients have at least one of these prior heart disease risk factors: high cholesterol, high blood pressure, diabetes, or cigarette use. For Elvira, a diabetes diagnosis was warning enough. Faced with medical risks that claimed the lives of a brother and sister, she snapped into action. Priorities shifted and she made significant changes in lifestyle and exercise. Not everyone has such clear, genetic confirmation of the threat. Without that direct connection, it's tempting to brush aside early indicators of heart risk. But when the heart sends notice that something is wrong, it's a message that goes to the core, shaking assumptions and prompting a reassessment of values. Heart disease and other life-threatening conditions often lead to a psychological "change of heart."

One of the first changes that many heart disease survivors initiate is a change in exercise patterns. Commonly, coronary patients are encouraged to participate in hospital-based cardiac rehabilitation programs that offer valuable assistance in making the transition into a more active, healthy life. But it isn't only heart patients who benefit from the physical and emotional rehabilitation an exercise program provides. Exercise delivers both prevention and remedy for survivors of almost any kind of medical or emotional trauma.

On the walks you have been taking these weeks, you've already experienced how movement can strengthen your physical body. This week's walks will expand that focus with exercises that can help you boost the cardiovascular benefits of your walks. But your walks have also been exercising your metaphorical heart—the heart we mean when we talk of getting to the core, or most meaningful aspect of a situation. It's the heart that sometimes "breaks" when things don't go as planned. It's the heart we call on for strength and faith when we "take heart."

Any event that jars mind or body creates a need for healing that goes beyond physical recovery and repair. When author Jean Shinoda Bolen, MD, writes about the psychological changes that attend serious illness or injury, she identifies the issues that spur transformations and changes for many people as "soul questions." They are questions that delve into personal truths and values. Questions that ask: Has my life had value? Do I matter? What unfinished business or dreams still call me? Illness opens the potential for changes and fresh commitment to personal values, she says in *Close to the Bone*.[2]

Healing the spiritual, symbolic heart is often a fundamental companion to healing physical wounds. Walking stirs circulation in mind and body, allowing wounds to heal. Move the muscles and the heart pumps with new vigor. Get things flowing and a hard heart may soften. A heavy heart can lighten. Maybe not quickly, but gradually, slowly, healing emerges in those moments when a current of fresh air and fresh fuel opens clogged passageways of our being.

In the year that followed my breast cancer diagnosis, my life tumbled through bumpy cycles of soul searching. Some days my heart was in my throat. Sometimes it opened wide. As I approached the sixth of eight aggressive chemotherapy treatments, scheduled at three-week intervals, my journal reveals changes that surprised even me.

Human adaptability is an amazing thing. Of course, I've known that about other people, but to observe this spirit of survival and accommodation in myself somehow surprises me. To adjust to a cycle that throws life off balance and then requires a steady, gentle return to stability in time to be knocked off-center again—how could anyone find that normal? And yet, I feel quite ordinary much of the time just now. Often, I even feel happy.

Is it "OK" to be happy when you have breast cancer? Not happy about cancer—happy in spite of cancer? Am I doing something wrong? Not digging deep enough? Not looking under and behind? I ask myself whether cancer destroys a wonderful life. Or is it possible that cancer will somehow turn out to be another charm? I don't know the answer yet. I do know that I have a deeper appreciation for my friends, my husband, and the community of support around me. I do know that I am loved.

The experience of finding myself loved, in spite of vulnerability or perhaps because of vulnerability, reshaped my identity. It gave me a new sense of security and a vocabulary shared by survivors of other life-changing events and illnesses. It is a vocabulary of amazement and gratitude. Disaster gives way to a healing of the heart.

A Path with Heart

It could be heart disease, or diabetes, or disability that brought you to a crossroads in life. It could be depression, divorce, cancer, or grief that stripped some choices from your reach and stretched an unfamiliar road before you. Faced with changes beyond control, we look for places to hold on. We look for choices we can still make. Sometimes a choice begins with mental preparation. We research options and outcomes. We study resources and ask questions. Then, as we ponder the possibilities, we may seek the wisdom of the heart. How does this choice feel? Where does it register in my body? How does it settle with my heart?

Look at every path closely and deliberately, writes Carlos Castaneda. "Then ask the question: Does this path have a heart? A path without heart is never enjoyable. On the other hand, a path with heart is easy; it does not make you work at liking it."[3]

Does this path have a heart? Who wouldn't seek such a route? A path of ease? A route of enjoyment? Castaneda's engaging question has inspired book titles and workshop descriptions. But for me, there's something lacking. This description of "heart" is not inclusive enough for the network of paths that have woven the fabric of my life, and perhaps of yours.

Every path has a heart! A path with heart may be warm and open. It might be cold and hard. A path with heart is vast and wide, as varied as the hearts we carry with us. One day you walk with a joyful heart, the next day a fearful one. Brave heart, broken heart, healthy heart, lonely heart. We meet them all on life's journey. The key lies in honoring the heart we encounter on each path. Soft or hard. Cold or warm. It changes as we change, moves as we move.

When I was writing *The Spirited Walker,* I interviewed a man who had walked 500 miles on the historic Camino de Santiago de Compostela pilgrimage trail in northern Spain. Since the Middle Ages, pilgrims have traveled this historic road, or *camino,* to the cathedral in Santiago where bones of the apostle James are said to rest. Early pilgrims who sought dispensation of sins with the walk established a tradition that continues today as travelers pause at churches and sacred sites along the way to obtain a village stamp confirming their passage. On arrival in Santiago, pilgrims apply at the cathedral for the *compostela,* an official document acknowledging completion of the pilgrimage. With the *compostela* comes forgiveness of sins, or release from suffering, for those who subscribed to the historic theology of this path.

James Carse undertook the trek, not to honor the bones of St. James, but as a tribute to his late wife. He wanted time to reflect on the path the two had shared through thirty-seven years of marriage. "I had gone to think things over, and instead, I didn't think at all," he told me.[4] "It was cleansing in a surprising way. From these efforts you get things you couldn't have imagined anyway."

His experience fed my curiosity about this pilgrimage trail that has enjoyed renewed popularity with long-distance walkers, tour companies, and hardy travelers from around the world. As I emerged from the physical and emotional upheaval of breast cancer a few years later, I wanted to celebrate the strength returning to my body, and to give thanks for spiritual and physical healing. I wanted a cleansing pilgrimage of my own. Rather than tackle the full 500-mile trek from the border of France to the west coast of Spain, I settled for an abbreviated version of the pilgrimage, a camino "sampler" that combined fourteen days of walking with intermittent days of travel by bus and train to bypass sections of the path.

With my husband in the lead, I set out on foot from Pamplona with an eager heart. The rocky path was slippery that morning after a rainy night. By the end of the day, I could feel the heat of blisters forming on my feet. I blamed it on unsteady footing. These boots had carried me many miles in the past without a single problem. By the second evening, full-blown sores flared on both feet. Eager heart turned to heavy heart as my hopes for a smooth, contemplative expedition faded. Reluctantly, we abandoned plans for a third day of walking and took a taxi twelve miles to our next destination.

A day of rest in the village of Santo Domingo de la Calzada gave my feet a break and allowed for leisurely exploration of the cathedral and the adjacent pilgrims' museum. As I browsed the displays of pilgrimage memorabilia, a passage caught my attention: "There are no pilgrimages without trails, branches, crossroads, and encounters with dung on the path. Without openness, without curiosity, without the capacity for surprise, there is no pilgrim. This is the glory of the journey and the motivation of the pilgrim."

I read it several times, working out an English translation of the words in the display case. My heart began to lift. Yes! Three days out and already the trail had led to surprises and encounters with unpleasantness. Here was confirmation, in the words of a previous pilgrim—openness to these intrusions and uncertainties is a mark of a true pilgrim!

We set out again, my feet cushioned in bandages, heading west through vineyards of the Rioja region. On the path, we learned to nod as villagers and farm workers greeted us. *"Buen camino,"* they called, wishing us a good journey. "Buen camino" announced cyclists who rolled past us on the trail. "Buen camino," we said to walkers from around the world with whom we shared a goal and these two words.

As the days passed and my feet healed, my heart grew light and playful. The traditional pilgrim's greeting morphed into a song, transforming the lilting notes of "Frère Jacques" into an opportunity for more Spanish practice. *"Buen camino, perigrino. Donde vas? Donde vas? Voy a Santiago, por mi compostela. Adios, Adios."* Round and round it danced lightly in my head. "Good journey, pilgrim. Where are you going? I'm going to Santiago, for my pilgrimage certificate. Farewell." The song delivered an antidote to discomfort and affirmed the goal at the end.

Our hopscotch journey to Santiago provided more than 120 miles of walking, putting us well above the 100 kilometer minimum required for satisfaction of the *compostela*. My Protestant upbringing had instilled in me no particular reverence for saints or dispensations. What lured me to the Camino de Santiago was not peace in the afterlife but peace in the present—the tranquility that comes with long walks. Still, the *compostela* document at the end would mark achievement of a goal. Like centuries of pilgrims before us, we stopped in village churches, opening up our pilgrimage "passports" to collect stamps as souvenirs.

As the trail neared Avila, I settled into the quiet rhythm of my steps and memorized a prayer by St. Teresa of Avila, founder of the contemplative order of Carmelite nuns. Journalism had provided opportunity to forge a warm friendship and respect for members of the order, and we maintained connection long after they allowed me to witness and write about callings and challenges of a religious vocation for contemporary women. On the path, St. Teresa's words provided both contemplative focus and practical distraction.

Nada te turbe,
Nada te espante,
Todo se pasa,
Dios no se muda.
La paciencia todo lo alcanza.
Quien a Dios tiene nada le falta.
Soló Dios basta!

May nothing disturb you,
May nothing astonish you,
Everything passes,
God does not change.
Patience can attain anything.
Who has God within, lacks nothing.
Only God is enough!

Through the high wheat fields beyond León, and into the muddy farmyards near Sarria, the words of St. Teresa and the rhythms of "Buen Camino, Perigrino" bumped around in my mind, sometimes colliding with complaints about the heat, my pack, or my feet. Sometimes settling into meditation. My heart opened to gratitude . . . gratitude for courage, for fortitude, and for the tender shoots of confidence growing in my cells as cancer eased out of the immediate present and into history.

At Palas de Rey, we caught a bus, as planned, avoiding several kilometers of roadside trekking through the industrial outskirts of Santiago. In the city, we dropped our packs at an inn and headed for the cathedral. "Buen camino," we said, as we joined a long line of pilgrims waiting to receive the *compostela* of completion. We inched forward for perhaps an hour to the desk where a clerk reviewed our pilgrimage credentials, checking village stamps and confirming distances we'd traveled on the route.

"You know the regulations?" she asked, a look of concern spreading across her face.

"Oh, yes," I assured her. "One hundred kilometers minimum." Despair deepened on her brow.

"The rules are clear," she continued. The minimum for the *compostela* is 100 kilometers—but not just any kilometers of the trail. Pilgrims must journey at least the *final* 100 kilometers by foot, including entry into Santiago. Our documents lacked stamps from the last two churches on the pilgrims' path.

My heart sank. Suddenly I understood why the ranks of walkers had thickened in the last days of our travel. How had the others known these regulations? How had I not known? An icy chill glazed my heart. Gone were St. Teresa's words of comfort. ("Let nothing disturb you. Everything passes.") Banished was the calm tranquility of the pilgrim. How could the organizer of this trip have missed such an essential piece of information? Why had I trusted his guidance, and not researched the trip myself? My fury fell on my fellow pilgrim—my historian spouse who had studied the route and designed an itinerary that focused on segments with historic or cultural significance. The *compostela* hadn't been a goal until my footsteps delivered me to a destination I had not seen coming.

The depth of my response stunned me. In the evening mass that welcomes pilgrims, my rage softened into grief. I sobbed through the blessings and the swirling incense. Tears seasoned a paella dinner, eaten in awkward silence. As we boarded a plane the following day to return home, I plotted how and when I could come back. It seemed imperative that I finish the walk in compliance with the rules. The grief in my heart had shifted to resentment. I'd have to do this myself to get it right!

Gradually, in retelling the story and bemoaning my fate to friends at home, my heart began to soften. Time and distance loosened my grip on the pain at the end of the trek. As I stepped back, my memory widened to include the glorious view from our room in a monastery where we spent a peaceful night. And the woman from Madrid, walking for a week of her vacation, who shared blister pads with me. The amiable church guides who welcomed us at each stop along the path. The companion who had embraced this journey because he embraced me.

When I saw the walk whole, as a journey greater than the destination, a gradual transformation emerged—an unnoticed shift from tourist to pilgrim. I returned to my notebook and read the lines I'd copied early in the journey: "There are no pilgrimages without trails, branches, crossroads, and encounters with dung on the path. Without openness, without curiosity, without the capacity for surprise, there is no pilgrim. This is the glory of the journey and the motivation of the pilgrim."

By the time we reached Santiago de Compostela, I had forgotten: It's not a rubber-stamped certificate that motivates a pilgrim. It's not a cathedral clerk who confers merit to the trek. Motivation springs from curiosity and from willingness to risk detour and surprise. It arises from openness to exploration of landscapes within and without. Just as James Carse had advised me: "From these efforts you get things you couldn't have imagined."

As I viewed the journey from a distance, heartache gave way to acceptance. The pull to return lost its force. This pilgrimage had reached its destination. It was clear, from here, that I'd walked a path with heart. A pilgrim's path with oh-so-many hearts.

SIDE STEPS: *Walking and Heart Health*

It's tempting to blame a desk job, long commute, or the conveniences of modern life for the lack of movement we get in day-to-day activities. After all, we can do library research without getting up from the computer, change television channels without leaving the couch, and purchase lunch at a drive-up window. Exercise is no longer a by-product of normal life for most of us. It takes commitment—a willful effort—to satisfy the body's need for exercise. Sometimes it takes a crisis.

No matter what form of healing may have motivated you to start walking, your steps are doing your heart a favor. Research consistently points to walking as a way to lower cholesterol, blood pressure, weight, and risk of heart disease. An inactive lifestyle is second only to cigarette smoking as a risk factor for heart disease.

Even short walks lead to healthy benefits for your heart. For overweight women in a study at Louisiana State University, just ten minutes daily of treadmill walking produced rapid health improvements.[5] More, of course, is better, but start where you can. Add an hour of gardening a week, and you get additional cardiac benefits. A University of Washington study demonstrated that people who regularly work in their gardens lower the risk of cardiac arrest by 66 percent, compared to people who do no exercise.[6]

As you become stronger, adding length and intensity to your walks increases cardiovascular health and weight loss. Exercise guidelines issued by the U.S. Department of Health and Human Services in 2009 recommend at least two and a half hours of moderate exercise a week for healthy adults. The exercise guidelines are based on a review of scientific research about physical activity and health.

"There was so much evidence of the benefits of physical activity," said Tufts University professor Miriam Nelson, who served on the review panel. "It's hard to believe more people don't realize this. People have to wake up."[7]

Some of you are already meeting or exceeding the recommended two and a half hours of exercise a week. Some are approaching that as you gradually extend the length of your walks. To comply with the government's definition of moderate exercise, you should be walking with enough energy to raise your heart rate a bit. The pace will depend on your present fitness level, but should require more exertion than a stroll. You can tell when you reach a moderate level of exercise by paying attention to how you feel. If you've been in a fitness center in recent years, you've probably seen a wall chart outlining levels of "perceived exertion." The chart ranks intensity levels from one to ten on a scale ranging from "very, very light" to "very, very hard." When you rank your effort at three to five on a scale of ten, you are very likely walking at a moderate level of effort. For most people, the aerobic exercise zone falls between five and seven on the perceived exertion scale. This is the range of effort to strive for to obtain maximum benefits for cardiac health. Build up slowly as you add length or intensity. Allow muscles to warm up before pushing for a brisk pace.

A pedometer offers another interesting method for assessing the intensity of your walks. Researchers have determined that an average rate of 100 steps per minute corresponds with moderate intensity for walkers who do not have physical limitations.[8] At that pace, a thirty-minute walk should produce a pedometer reading of 3,000 steps. A twenty-minute walk nets 2,000 steps. Although pedometer readings may not be precise, they add another source of feedback and information that can strengthen a walking habit, and also strengthen your heart. Try it out with a ten-minute walk test to see how your pace measures up to the suggested goal. If you end up within 50 steps up or down from 1,000 steps in ten minutes, you're walking in the target range and will have traveled about a half mile.

Don't be dismayed if you are not able to meet the recommended amount of exercise or the intensity levels suggested. And above all, don't give up. Any exercise is better than none. The American Heart Association estimates that adults gain about two hours of life expectancy for each hour they spend in a regular exercise activity.[9] Inactivity is the most risky choice you can make when it comes to the health of your heart.

TOOL TALK: *Pedometer Basics*

If you have a pedometer tucked in a drawer someplace, this is the time to dig it out. For people who love information, pedometers can boost motivation. If you don't already have a pedometer, consider purchasing an inexpensive model, or check to see if your health insurance company, employer, or the local hospital has pedometers to give away. Many organizations provide pedometers as a fitness incentive. Research has demonstrated that walkers who wear pedometers regularly get more exercise daily than walkers who do not.[10]

Choose a simple model if you buy a pedometer. All you really need to know is how many steps you are taking. Unless you are a serious techie, calculations about distance walked and calories burned simply add confusion and complications.

Put the pedometer on your waistband, positioning it in line with your kneecap. Do not put it in your pocket, on a beltloop, or on a jacket. Basic pedometers are simply pendulums. They "count" your steps by registering the up and down movement of your hips as you walk. Because we have different walking styles and strides, you may have to experiment with the best position on your waist. Test the accuracy of the pedometer by setting it to zero and then counting off twenty or thirty steps. Check the pedometer and see if it agrees with your count. If you are within two or three steps, that's close enough. If you are way off, try moving the pedometer a bit more to the outside of your hip. Test again. If that doesn't improve accuracy, try moving the pedometer on the waistband closer to the center of your stomach. Keep inching it around your waist until you get a fairly accurate count. If you have an ample stomach, you may find that you get the truest count by placing the pedometer at the back of your waistband rather than in the front.

Once you get the pedometer positioned, what does it tell you? The most important information is the number of steps you take on an average day. Put the pedometer on in the morning and let it track your steps through a full day. Wear it at work. At the grocery store. Walking the dog. Taking out the garbage. If you work as a nurse or waiter or gardener, you may exceed 20,000 steps a day. But most of us register fewer than 5,000 steps as we move through the routines of daily life. After wearing the pedometer for a few days, you will have a baseline measurement for your own daily average.

Many organizations promote the popular recommendation that people strive to take an average of 10,000 steps a day, or 70,000 steps a week, for basic health and fitness. In order to meet that recommendation, most people need to schedule exercise beyond routine activity. As you continue this walking program, you might move gradually toward the goal of 70,000 steps a week. Seek to increase your steps no more than 10 percent a week so that you build strength and endurance, both physically and mentally.

Even the most basic step-counter pedometer can give you feedback on distance and time walked, if you're content with averages. A stride length of two-and-a-half feet is considered to be an average stride for adult walkers. With that average, 2,000 steps makes one mile. It's a rough estimate, but close enough to give you a sense of achievement.

Of course, "average" is a loose term. Your own stride length changes frequently. The steps you take from the bedroom to the kitchen are probably different from your stride on a neighborhood sidewalk. It changes when you climb a set of steps or move onto a rocky trail instead of an asphalt path. But in all of those situations you are still taking steps, and movement is what matters when you are measuring exercise.

If you want to play with pedometer readings, start with these numbers based on an average stride length of two-and-a-half feet.

At a moderate walking pace of 20 minutes per mile:

    500 steps = about ¼ mile = about 5 minutes
    1,000 steps = about ½ mile = about 10 minutes
    2,000 steps = about 1 mile = about 20 minutes

At a brisk walking pace of 15 minutes per mile:

    625 steps = about ⅓ mile = about 5 minutes
    1,250 steps = about ⅔ mile = about 10 minutes
    2,000 steps = about 1 mile = about 15 minutes

The purpose of life is to increase the warm heart.

—Dalai Lama

When you put your heart into a project, or a challenge, it means you give it your all—an emotional commitment fuels your efforts. A successful exercise program also requires an emotional commitment. You may begin a fitness routine for lots of good reasons—exercise is important to health, you know you should be doing it, and so on. But when you find a form of exercise that feeds your emotional heart, as well as your physical heart, your efforts become a labor of love. Yes, exercise is still a labor at times, but it's an effort that satisfies your spirit.

This week's walks give you an opportunity to put your whole heart into your exercise rotation. Cardiovascular health isn't essential to emotional healing, and probably isn't the primary reason you have been following the eight-week Walking Well program. If you have a heart condition or physical challenges that limit your ability to walk faster, or to push the intensity level of your exercise, don't attempt the Aerobic Heart Intervals out-lined this week. Choose the alternative Compassionate Heart walk instead.

If you are physically and mentally ready to pick up the pace, you'll find it easier if you make a few adjustments in your stride. When you want to walk faster, it helps to shorten your stride a bit. Short steps enable you to have faster turnover from foot to foot. Arms add momentum. Bend your arms at the elbow, into a ninety-degree angle, and use them to set your pace. You'll discover that when you increase the speed with which you swing the arms, your feet will follow. Keep shoulders relaxed and posture erect to facilitate full, regular breathing.

For most walkers, the greatest obstacle to an aerobic pace is mental readiness. Pacing begins in the mind, with a clear intention to accelerate enough to increase heart rate and breathing rhythm. Typically, people identify this level as "somewhat hard."

On an exertion scale of one to ten, it's usually between four and seven. Exercising at this level once or twice a week benefits cardiac health and improves overall fitness. But I've found it also benefits the mind. When you pick up the pace, your mind will protest: "This is hard. I don't want to do this today." That mental complaining signals that you've reached the "somewhat hard" level. Your effort then is no longer automatic—it takes cooperation of brain and body to sustain it. This is when you need cognitive override to block the complaints. Bring body and mind together by counting steps or chanting. Create a cadence of *In-two-three, Out-two-three*. Or sing "Yankee Doodle Dandy" to yourself. Use the focusing techniques you've been learning these past weeks to carry you through the initial resistance that always emerges when you move beyond your comfort zone.

1. AEROBIC HEART INTERVALS

Short intervals of fast walking help you build stamina and cardiovascular health. By doing intervals, you raise heart rate for a set time or distance and then slow down to a normal pace for an equal time. The slow-down phase is a recovery period that brings heart rate and breathing back to a steady rate. Always do intervals after five minutes of warm-up walking so your muscles are warm and ready to work. You reduce the risk of injury when you do intervals because your body adjusts to the increases with a cycle of repetitions.

Start with a series of three interval cycles. Pick up the pace so that you're moving with energy and a sense of urgency. Get your arms in the act to help. Count fifty steps. Then relax and continue walking at a normal pace for fifty steps. Repeat fifty steps of increased effort and fifty steps of recovery for three full cycles. That's it. The counting helps keep your mind busy and helps you stay focused.

Walking Well isn't meant to be a fitness program; it's a healing program. Intervals are a way to encourage mind-body cooperation. If you are strong and fit, expand the length or number of intervals as you desire. Don't feel that intervals are essential if you are not ready for this effort. You can come back to this exercise as you grow stronger.

2. BUNGEE CORD INTERVALS

It's easy to do a variety of intervals by putting on the imaginary bungee cord that you learned to use in Week Four. Set a visual target a short distance ahead of you and hook your bungee cord to the goal. In a residential neighborhood, you might target a curbside tree and let the pull of the bungee cord increase your walking pace until you feel you are walking "somewhat hard." Recover with a normal pace for an equal distance before resetting the cord on another tree. The variation of speed and focus that intervals provide helps jump-start energy when you are feeling lethargic or bored on a walk. The change of pace infuses your cells with oxygen.

3. COMPASSIONATE HEART ALTERNATIVE

If you are not physically ready for a faster walking pace, replace the Aerobic Heart Intervals or Bungee Cord Intervals on the weekly guides below with this Compassionate Heart variation on a loving kindness meditation. The pattern is similar to Yin-Yang Breath.

1. Imagine you have energy receptors in the arches of your feet, sort of like vacuum openings that draw energy up from the earth. Feel the strong pull as you inhale love up through your feet and draw it up into your heart. Let your heart open and fill with loving energy. As you exhale, imagine all that love spilling out the top of your head and washing back down over your own body, a cloak of acceptance, peace, and compassion. Repeat several times, inhaling love through your feet and then letting it flow down from the top of your head as you exhale.

2. When you feel filled with love, change the exhalation a bit. Inhale love as before and then exhale it out to someone you care for. Imagine that person as you exhale loving kindness, peace, and compassion. Repeat this cycle several times.

3. Let your love spread even farther as you exhale love to all the people on the street where you are walking, or into the atmosphere wherever you are. Let your breath be a prayer of peace and compassion, spreading out to the world around you. Then inhale love through your feet, refilling your own heart with loving energy.

Previous Exercises You'll Use This Week

1. BREATHE IN, BREATHE OUT (WEEK ONE)

Mentally remind yourself *In* as you inhale and *Out* as you exhale. Focusing on words and breath speeds the release of stress.

2. FOUR-STEP: IN-2-3-4 CADENCE (WEEK TWO)

Create a four-count cadence of feet and breath by mentally repeating *In-two-three-four, Out-two-three-four* as you inhale and exhale. Four steps for each inhalation. Four steps for each exhalation.

3. THREE-STEP: IN-2-3 CADENCE (WEEK THREE)

Mentally repeat to yourself, *In-two-three, Out-two-three* so you set the rhythm in your mind as well as with your breath and feet. Be aware that your lead foot alternates on this odd-number count. If you say *In* on the right foot, you'll say *Out* on the left foot.

4. MENTAL MARINADES (WEEK THREE)

Using the rhythm of either the four-count or the three-count cadence, repeat a mental marinade that supports your well-being. Starters might be:

> I am strong, Yes, I am
> I am here, I am whole
> Life is good, I give thanks
> I am walking, I am breathing
> I am walking, I am healing

4. IMAGINE: SMOOTH AND TALL (WEEK FOUR)

Mentally repeat *I am smooth, I am tall,* to create a three-count cadence. As you say *smooth* in your mind, imagine your foot is a rocker, landing on the heel and rolling through to the toe with each step. As you say *tall,* imagine a cord extending from the top of your head to a trolley line overhead, holding you erect. Breathe and glide!

5. LOVE IN, FEAR OUT (WEEK FOUR)

Use the three-count cadence for this exercise, mentally saying *Love comes in* as you inhale. As you exhale, say *Fear goes out.* Imagine love coming in with each breath. Feel love filling your lungs and heart. As you exhale, think of flushing limiting fears out of your cells, releasing them into the air.

6. SAY THANK YOU (WEEK ONE)

End each walk with a moment of appreciation for your body, your neighborhood, your family, your friends, your opportunities to give and receive love.

Week Seven Goals Overview

Walk Level	Walk Time Goal	Silent Segment Time Goal
Stepping Out	Walk 6 days 18–22 min. a day	10 min. silent
Mid-Stride	Walk 6 days 25 min. 4–5 days 30 min. 1–2 days	15–20 min. silent
Strong and Steady	Walk 6 days 30 min. 4–5 days 40 min. 1–2 days	20–30 min. silent

Week Seven Daily Walk Guidelines

Rotate walks at your level for variety during the week. Try walks at a different level if you want more or less exercise. You are always welcome to extend walks when you are feeling energetic. Add in a previous focus technique you have enjoyed, or extend the time for these suggested focus tools.

Compassionate Heart Alternative
Replace Aerobic Segment: Love In, Love Out

Stepping Out		
Week 7	Focusing Techniques Rotate routines for variety	Suggested Timing

2 days
18–22 min.
	1. Three-Step:
	   In-2-3 Cadence
	2. Mental Marinades:
	   Three-Step Cadence
	3. Say Thank You
		10 min.
		
		10 min.
		
		2 min.

2 days 18–22 min.	1. Breathe In, Breathe Out Or: Walk, Talk, Listen 2. Imagine: Smooth and Tall 3. Bungee Cord Intervals 4. Say Thank You	10 min. 5 min. 5 min. 2 min.

2 days
18–22 min.
	1. Four-Step:
	   In-2-3-4 Cadence
	2. Mental Marinades:
	   Four-Step Cadence
	3. Say Thank You
		10 min.
		
		10 min.
		
		2 min.

Mid-Stride		
Week 7	**Focusing Techniques** Rotate routines for variety	**Suggested Timing**

4–5 days
25 min.
	1. Three-Step:
	   In-2-3 Cadence
	   Or: Walk, Talk, Listen
	2. Imagine: Smooth and Tall
	3. Aerobic Heart Intervals
	   Or: Bungee Cord Intervals
	4. Say Thank You
		10 min.
		
		5 min.
		8 min.
		
		2 min.

1–2 days
30 min.
	1. Breathe In, Breathe Out
	   Or: Walk, Talk, Listen
	2. Four-Step:
	   In-2-3-4 Cadence
	3. Mental Marinades
	4. Say Thank You
		10 min.
		
		8 min.
		
		10 min.
		2 min.

Strong and Steady		
Week 7	**Focusing Techniques** Rotate routines for variety	**Suggested Timing**

4–5 days
30 min.
	1. Love In, Fear Out
	2. Four-Step:
	   In-2-3-4 Cadence
	3. Mental Marinades:
	   Four-Step Cadence
	4. Say Thank You
		10 min.
		8 min.
		
		10 min.
		
		2 min.

1–2 days
40 min.
	1. Breathe In, Breathe Out
	   Or: Walk, Talk, Listen
	2. Three-Step:
	   In-2-3 Cadence
	3. Imagine: Smooth and Tall
	4. Aerobic Heart Intervals
	   Or: Bungee Cord Intervals
	5. Say Thank You
		10 min.
		
		10 min.
		
		8 min.
		10 min.
		
		2 min.

Log In

Reinforce your walking practice by noticing what made your walk significant. Record your walking time, your route, and thoughts on the walking log for Week Seven.

- Are you feeling stronger physically in your walks?
- Are you noticing changes in your energy level after walks?
- How did it feel to push yourself to a faster pace?
- What goes on in your mind when you speed up?
- What focusing technique did you enjoy most? Why?
- Did you find a miracle as you walked? What was it?
- How did it feel to shower yourself, and others, in love?
- What are you thankful for today?

By paying attention to these things, you continue to learn what motivates and energizes you when you walk.

Week Eight

A Healthy Habit

Habits give us more than structure—they reflect values and hopes. Patterns of exercise, sleep, eating, work, and hygiene lend daily support to ideals that give our lives meaning. In times of crisis, healthy habits provide a framework to lean on. This week, create a format that integrates the tools you have learned in an enduring habit.

*D*anny Foto held his two-year-old son in his arms as he stood on the doorstep of his home in a New Orleans suburb and watched for the morning school bus that would pick up his two daughters. The girls waited at the curb. When a car sped down the residential street, Danny recognized the driver as the adult son of a neighbor. "Slow down," Danny shouted, as the speeding car careened into the driveway next door. Then he turned his focus back to his daughters at the curb.

Court records reveal that the driver had a history of mental illness and had recently been fighting with his parents. Still no one imagined the unimaginable until he emerged from the home with a twelve-gauge shotgun and fired three blasts into the neighborhood. One shot killed Danny instantly. Another wounded his young son. The third shattered the ankle of a neighbor watching from across the street.

"During that awful time in my life, I was numb," Danny's mother recalls five years after the shooting.[1] "It was horrible. My walking buddy said, 'Whatever you want to do, we will do. If you want to walk, talk, stroll . . . we will do it.'"

Karen Foto wanted to walk. And she wanted to talk. Danny, the eldest of her three grown children, was thirty-nine at the time of his death. His young son survived the attack. "I needed people around me," Karen says. "I needed to vent. It was due to mental illness and there's nothing you can do about it. So the walking, and being able to talk, gave me relief. I needed to do both."

Long before tragedy pumped urgency into her steps, Karen had been a walker. "I think my husband pushed me into walking, with his love of nature," she says. Family vacations with three young children brought road trips to national parks, with hikes for recreation. "I began to fall in love with nature." At home, walks on the two-mile walking loop in a neighborhood park drew nature into Karen's daily life. As a registered nurse who walked the halls of a New Orleans hospital, it wasn't exercise as much as renewal that she sought on her outings. "At that time, with three kids at home and being a nurse, getting away for a walk was my release," she says. "Mostly I walked alone. I wanted quiet time. I wanted to meditate or pray."

When their children were grown, Karen and her husband moved from New Orleans to a community on the north shore, across Lake Pontchartrain. A major attraction of the area, she says, is the three-mile walking path that loops through the housing division where they settled. "I can walk out my back door and be on the trail. I feel like I am walking in my own park."

When Karen returned to her nursing position one month after her son's death, she resumed the daily lunch walks shared with a group of nursing colleagues. From the hospital, they could circle the Super Dome or retreat to a nearby mall to walk the corridors in foul weather. The walks, she says, helped keep her afloat in a flood of grief.

A year had passed when tragedy struck again. A diagnosis of breast cancer unleashed a fresh wave of uncertainty and fear for Karen. She tackled the intruder straight on with surgery, radiation, and walking. Gradually, life stabilized, although the pain of back-to-back disasters trailed behind her like a shadow. The shadow lengthened the following year when newscasters issued warnings of a major storm approaching New Orleans. As alarm grew about the intensity of Hurricane Katrina, Karen and her husband gathered up children and grandchildren and evacuated to Mississippi. For two weeks, they lived together in hotel rooms and waited for news. Karen's north shore home was spared. Danny's family was not as fortunate. Floodwaters reached the second story of their house, destroying photos and cherished mementos of the man who had died just two years earlier.

For six months, displaced family members camped out at Karen's home while making recovery efforts at their own homes. "We had a house that wasn't flooded, so we took others in," she says. "That was the norm down here. If you had a house, you just opened your doors. It's amazing what people did."

With life in turmoil, Karen took a familiar path. She turned to the walking trail behind her house and found comfort in an established habit. "I find that I do my best thinking when I am walking," she says. "I feel like I'm an addict and exercise is the perfect drug for me. I just feel good when I do it, and when I don't do it, I miss it. It's both a physical health and emotional health exercise, that's what it is."

When I met Karen, about five years after her son's death and two years after Hurricane Katrina, she had signed up as a volunteer leader for a healing walks program being introduced at a community hospital near her. Without walking, she insists, she's not sure how she could have endured the rapid-fire sequence of three major, life-shaking tragedies in as many years. She might have given up, she says, but for the power of her four Fs—family, friends, faith, and feet.

I would expand the alphabet to include a capital H for habit. Because Karen had established a habit of lunchtime walks with coworkers, she had a structure in place that helped keep her moving when hard times tripped her. Because she had learned to value silent walks of prayer and meditation on the path behind her home, she had a familiar, healing retreat.

You're creating the same safety net with the walks you've been taking. With the power of habit to sustain momentum, you can regain footing more readily when life delivers a harsh blow. Include family, friends, and faith in the habit, and the structure of support grows even stronger.

Habit Forming

If you've been following the Walking Well program for seven weeks, you're establishing a pattern that can ease you into a habit. If you've noticed that walking brings improvements in mood, energy, or fitness, you've picked up incentives that add impetus. When your steps produce direct results in energy, alertness, or mood, the benefits supply motivation. Some sources say it takes an average of three months to fully embrace a new habit. In that case, this eight-week walking program has guided you two-thirds of the way. If you were a former exerciser who lost momentum, you may have restored a stable exercise pattern by now.

Attitude is one of the keys to sustaining any new behavior. If you feel that your action serves a purpose—that it contributes to an outcome you consider valuable—you are more likely to stick with it. When her children were young, Karen Foto's daily walks served an important purpose of providing time to regroup and reconnect with herself amid the demands of nursing and her life as a wife and mother. The physical benefits were secondary; Karen sought renewal of mind and spirit in her walks. Later, when her children were grown, Karen moved into an administrative position at the hospital, and the purpose of her walks shifted. Physical exercise became her motivation. Then, when tragedy shook the framework of her life, she walked for yet another purpose. She walked to heal. She walked to pray. She walked to feel the stability of habit—to travel a familiar path in a time of uncertainty.

Knowing *why* you are exercising helps you stick to your goals, says Diane Doster, an exercise scientist who develops wellness programs for people contending with Parkinson's disease, cancer, osteoporosis, diabetes, and the limitations of aging. Often people approach exercise as a *should*—everyone *should* exercise. But *shoulds* are a burden, not a reason. Doster encourages clients to back up and ask a series of *why* questions when they embark on a lifestyle change.

"If a person comes to me and wants to lose weight, I'll ask why," Doster says.[2] If the response is that a physician recommended it, that's not enough. That might get you started, but it won't carry you through energy slumps or schedule disruptions. It's not enough to elicit personal commitment and satisfaction. It calls for further questions.

Do you agree with the doctor's recommendation? Why?

Is weight a health concern for you? Why?

Does weight prevent you from doing things you want to do?

Eventually, the questions lead to an emotional conviction—a personal purpose:

I want to lose weight so I can breathe better and get back to playing on the company softball team.

I want to lose weight to reduce knee strain so I can dance with my spouse for our anniversary.

For someone else, the initial reason for beginning an exercise program might be to improve balance and lessen the risk of falls. Again, Doster probes beyond balance to get to deeper *whys*.

Why do you need better balance?

Because I'm afraid of falling.

What will happen if you fall?

I might have to go to a nursing home or assisted living.

Why would that be a problem?

I don't want to leave my own home.

Why?

I want to be independent. I want to keep my cat.

Maybe the cat becomes the most important "why"—a purpose clear and personal enough that it gives meaning to activities that build stability and balance. With a clear purpose, you increase the odds of sticking with a resolution. Exercise becomes something you "want" to do, and not something you "should" do. It leads to an outcome you value. Get beyond "should" by asking "why," and the answer reveals a personal goal that gives your steps purpose and meaning.

This is a process you can do for yourself. Why are you walking? If you don't have an answer that is clear, personal, and linked to emotion as well as logic, ask yourself some questions:

- What purpose does walking serve in my life?
- What need does it satisfy? What goal does it help me achieve?
- Is my purpose emotional healing and stability?
- Mental clarity? Why is that important to me?
- Physical recovery and balance? Why do I want that?
- Do walks give me needed quiet time alone?
- Do they give me connection with nature?
- Do they provide interaction with friends?

Maybe the purpose will shift from day to day, or from year to year, as your needs change. But identifying what you desire from your walks will help you get it. Getting what you seek will keep you moving. "What keeps us going is that we experience results," Doster says. "Success might be that every time I exercise, I have a mood shift and my day is better, or I'm feeling stronger and more grounded after a walk. That's important. The rewards that come from what we are doing keep the habit going."

Rarely does anyone integrate a new habit by traveling a straight line, Doster warns. Be prepared for a path with twists and turns. "Ideally, we would all like to take the straight road," she says. "We would like to be efficient. But it's just part of being human to zigzag on the path. If you miss a day and don't walk, that's just a zigzag. It's not a failure. It's the personal conclusion that you have failed—'so why keep going?'—that leads to dropout with exercise. Allow yourself to be human, and be aware that it is always a choice to step back on the path. It's a zigzag path, and that's OK."

Exercise Your Writes

As a source of ongoing motivation, almost nothing beats a written walking log. A log gives you another form of results that you can see. It reminds you of the benefits you're finding. If you haven't been keeping track of your progress on this program, it's time to give it a try. You might begin with something as simple as a check mark on your calendar for every day that you walk. Remember, your walks are a form of medicine that is most effective when taken daily. The check mark is evidence that you got your daily-recommended dose of oxygen and circulation. If you take other medications regularly, think of walking as a prescription that you don't swallow but rather inhale.

People who take time to record information about their workouts typically have a higher rate of success in sticking with exercise programs. Perhaps that's because keeping a log reminds you why you are walking, and encourages you to notice what you gain from your effort. The log format for this program suggests that you pay attention to your mood, your energy level, and your environment as you walk. This week, you might ask yourself what it is you are seeking from these walks. Then, write that goal at the top of your log as a reminder. After each walk, make a quick note about the experience. If you miss a day, write down the reason. Perhaps you'll discover patterns that sabotage your exercise. When you know what your downfall is, you may be able to make changes that support you. Ask a friend to meet you for walks. Take five-minute walks instead of none when you don't have time for fifteen or thirty minutes.

Find ways to personalize your log. Perhaps you make a practice of recording one sensory observation from each walk. It might be a "miracle" of nature that caught your eye as you circled the block. Something you smelled, or heard, or felt. If your steps lead you to a healing prayer or affirmation, make a note of the words you found supportive or inspiring. Do you feel more energy or less at the end of the walk? If your energy or mood sags at the end of a walk, make a change. Vary the length or the route. Look for a walking group that would add social connection to the exercise.

When you experiment with an exercise change, record variations in your mood or energy in the log.

....

The knowledge that exercise has been beneficial in the past is the key to cognitive override—the secret weapon in the battle against inertia.

....

Your walking log is a personal research project. As you record data, you gather evidence of the influence walking has on your energy, mood, vitality, or personal sense of satisfaction. That evidence empowers you when it feels as if you can't get out of the chair. The knowledge that exercise has been beneficial in the past is the key to cognitive override—the secret weapon in the battle against inertia.

"If one is too tired to move, but you know, because you have done this before, that when you begin to walk you won't be as tired anymore, you can override the impulse not to exercise," says research psychologist Robert Thayer of California State University, Long Beach.[3] Everyone encounters challenges that threaten commitment. It's the weather, or work, or a medical appointment. It's a bad day, a bad mood, or a bad time.

"That's the day in and day out part of being human—the unruly mind that will try to sabotage exercise," says Doster. "Cognitive override is saying 'no' to that mental banter. It's saying, 'I'm not going to give in and lie on the couch. I'm going to get up because this is something I want to accomplish in my life.'"

From Crisis to Cause

A diagnosis of cancer at age forty-three jarred Carrie Wells's expectations of what she wanted from life. A New York City bank employee with a ten-year-old-daughter, a husband, and a high-rise city residence, she was on the way up in pursuit of bright dreams for her family and career. Cancer knocked the breath out of her. It stalled her momentum briefly, while she shifted from crisis to cause.

"I took a big turn in my life because of my diagnosis," she says.[4] "At first, I was at doctors' offices all the time, and I met people who carried this burden of cancer around. I don't know where it comes from, but they had turned into 'woe is me' people. I didn't want to be like that. So, there I was—no hair, no eyebrows—but I went out and bought my first pair of sneakers."

As a New Yorker, Carrie knew how to walk. Before cancer she had traveled the half-mile between her apartment and her work in business shoes. Cancer put new purpose in her steps. More than simply transportation to work, it became a means of reaching a goal. Carrie wanted to survive. She joined a clinical trial on meditation where participants learned visualization and breathing techniques to lower stress and enhance immune functions. Biofeedback machines revealed surprising results, she says. "I started out thinking I didn't believe in meditation, but I could see that meditation and visualization really did something to my body."

Then she started walking. "I'm not an exerciser by nature, but people said I needed exercise to build immune defenses," she explains. As soon as the physical healing from a mastectomy and reconstructive surgery permitted, she began supplementing her office walks with an hour of fitness walking at noon. As her strength returned, she added weekend walks that carried her into other neighborhoods around the city. She wanted to boost her odds of continued health. She wanted to live with enthusiasm.

"I had some depression at the beginning, yes, but walking brought me out of that," she says. "I discovered that walking strengthened my mind, my body, my spirit. It's the only time I am alone, in my head. It's meditation. I realize that was missing in my life before." By the time she could run her fingers through the fuzz of new hair, she had signed up to walk sixty miles in a three-day cancer benefit walk. As she trained for the event, new questions swirled in her wake. "I started asking, 'Now what am I going to do with my life?' I realized that every day is important."

One benefit walk led to another, and then another. Step by step, the cancer crisis that prompted Carrie's second look at life transformed itself into a cause. In the years since her 2002 diagnosis, she has walked hundreds of miles in benefit events, rallying friends and family to join her in the effort. She has raised thousands of dollars in support of cancer research, and now plays a role in determining how some of that money is spent. From walking for a cause, she advanced to reading for a cause, and became a survivor participant on the review panel that evaluates medical research grant requests for the Department of Defense. It is, she says, the hardest work she has ever done, and some of the most rewarding. In addition, she screens grant applications for the Susan G. Komen Breast Cancer Foundation and evaluates community service proposals for the Lance Armstrong Foundation.

"Cancer put me on track," she says. "I don't want to think about cancer as a good thing or a bad thing, but it gave me a place to contribute. I was already volunteering in the community, but the cancer diagnosis gave me a different road to travel." Cancer advocacy put new purpose in Carrie's life. "This is something I choose to do," she says. "I'm proud of myself when I finish those proposals."

And she continues to walk, sustaining a habit that took root in the passion and purpose she discovered at benefit walks. "Walking has given my life a rhythm, a pace," she says. "It's such a central part of my life now. It slows me down when I need that, and it speeds me up when I am feeling low energy or think that my life is boring. I'm so thankful for walking because that's where I put myself back together. It gave me the inner strength to do the advocacy work I thought was going to be important to make my life worthwhile."

Purpose-Driven Steps

Many national organizations serving victims of crisis encourage walking with community fundraising walks that attract millions of people each year. These events generate funds for research and support services, but equally important, they generate purpose and a sense of community for participants. Carrie's involvement in benefit walks triggered a deep commitment to giving back in appreciation for her own restored health. Benefit walks offer a good way to solidify or energize a walking habit.

Benefit events support more than physical healing and recovery. Often they facilitate emotional healing. They transform a tragic experience into a cause that has meaning. At the same time, they preserve connection to a situation that has shaken attitudes, safety, and goals. They link the past and the future. One moves on, taking positive action to help others, without abandoning memory of what has been lost or changed. Although it is not possible, and perhaps not even desirable, to eliminate the emotional pain of a traumatic experience, the ability to find some meaning in the tragedy sets in motion a transition from victim to survivor, says psychologist Donald Meichenbaum, whose work has focused on survivors of trauma. Rather than try to erase the emotional pain of a traumatic experience, seek to find some meaning in it, he advises.[5]

The founders of Mothers Against Drunk Driving (MADD) acted in passionate response to the tragic loss of a child by vowing to strengthen repercussions for drivers who ignore alcohol safety. They turned a crisis into a cause that preserves the memory of their loss, and still enables them to move forward, helping others. The Susan G. Komen Breast Cancer Foundation arose out of one woman's resolve to remember and honor her sister. It, like many other charitable organizations, now gives purpose to millions of other survivors who regain a hold on life by grasping a cause that supports research.

People progress from viewing themselves as victims, to survivors, and even thrivers, as they transform their pain into something that can help others, says Meichenbaum. "A thriver is someone who still remembers, but can use that pain more effectively."

SIDE STEPS: *Walking and Feet*

You can make all the plans and resolutions you want. Set goals. Sign up for fundraisers. Buy new shoes. But when it actually comes to walking your talk, it all depends on how you treat your feet. As you increase the length or frequency of your walks, it's wise to incorporate foot-care habits that will support you in reaching your goals.

Your feet are intricate, complicated structures. Each foot boasts twenty-six separate bones and thirty-three joints that must work together smoothly in order for you to take a step. Strong, healthy feet allow you to stay active. When you walk, run, play, dance, or stand at the stove to cook, your feet are subjected to stress. Even a minor complaint like a blister can disrupt walking patterns, throwing off your stride and your walking commitment.

You can protect your feet from many injuries by wearing the right shoes when you walk, and by strengthening and stretching muscles in your foot and ankle.

SHOES

Your feet swell during sustained walking, so shop for shoes late in the day, when your feet are likely to be swollen. Select a shoe that is half an inch longer than your foot and has a wide, high toe box, leaving plenty of room for your toes to move. Properly fitted walking shoes are likely to be one size larger than your dress shoes. Stroll around the showroom with the shoes on to test the fit before making a purchase.

STRETCH AND STRENGTHEN

Toe lifts help strengthen and stretch muscles in your ankles and arch. Stand on a level surface with your hands on the back of a straight-backed chair for balance. Rise up on your toes and hold the lift for a count of five. Lower and repeat. Work up to three sets of ten lifts daily.

Another version of toe lifts can be done sitting down. Lift one foot and alternately point the toes toward the ground and then toward your face. If you are barefoot, stretch your toes out wide as you raise the foot to increase flexibility. Repeat ten times with each foot.

ARCH SUPPORT

Gentle massage helps circulation in muscles and tendons of the arch, where tension builds on a long walk. When you are sitting down to watch television, give yourself a foot massage. Apply pressure with your thumb along the arch of the foot, and circle your toes to open up joints. If you prefer, stand up and rotate one foot on top of a tennis ball for a strong, energizing massage. Control how deep the massage goes by controlling how much weight you put on the tennis ball. Foot massage may help protect against the development of plantar fascitis, a painful heel irritation that can result from putting increased demand on your feet.

DIABETES AND NEUROPATHY

Diabetes causes elevated blood sugar levels, which can damage blood vessels and nerves in the body. Nerve damage results in a loss of feeling, or neuropathy, and increases risk of circulation problems and infection. Diabetes can also result in poor blood flow in the legs and feet, which slows the healing time for sores or wounds. Avoid problems with daily foot examinations to identify cuts or blisters that need treatment.

Some cancer treatment drugs, as well back injuries or back surgeries, also can cause the numbness of neuropathy. Stable shoes, walking sticks, and regular foot examinations make walking safer and more enjoyable. Toe numbness that occurs only when you walk is likely to be the result of shoes that are too small or laces that are too tight.

OSTEOARTHRITIS

Because the foot has thirty-three joints, it's not surprising that some of them suffer the inflammation that occurs with osteoarthritis. The big toe joint is the site most commonly affected. Ice packs, foot massage, and supportive shoes may help ease the swelling that causes pain.

BLISTERS

New shoes or long-distance walks can result in the painful swelling of blisters. Blisters are bubbles of fluid that form when the skin rubs against an irritant. Most blisters heal in a few days and can be protected with moleskin or cushioned bandages. A dab of lubricant, such as petroleum jelly, can reduce skin irritation to the area around a blister. Minimize the risk of blisters by choosing specially fabricated wicking socks that draw moisture away from the skin. If your feet sweat heavily, dust them with talcum powder before putting on socks.

BE VIGILANT

If you develop a foot problem that doesn't go away, or if you have pain that affects your walking posture and stride, get a professional assessment. When you try to accommodate a persistent problem on the foot, you risk compounding the trouble by triggering pain in a knee or hip.

Motivation is what gets you started.
Habit is what keeps you going.

—Jim Ryun, three-time Olympian

Good habits or bad habits form the same way—they grow out of repetition. Habits provide continuity and routines that maintain order in our lives. But "habit" is a loaded word for some people. It can trigger resistance both in those who hear the word as a demand for rigid discipline and in those who dismiss habits as mindless patterns of behavior. I like to think of my walking habit as a "practice." To call my walks a practice recognizes the role of repetition in shaping a skill or behavior, and it also honors the spiritual component of these walks. "Practice" acknowledges the intentionality of my walks. This pattern is not mindless— every walk represents a choice. Walking is something I value and choose on a regular basis. The spiritual centering I gain brings healing to the fragmentation of daily life. It is a habit, or a practice, for restoring wholeness and resourcefulness.

As you begin the eighth week of this walking program, you have probably begun to feel the rhythm of repetition as you fit walking into your routines. Some days it's easy, and some days a debate. You have to talk yourself into doing it. But as the practice grows more and more familiar, the pattern itself becomes a kind of motivation, restoring order and structure in your life. Eventually, it's the renewed energy, strength, and connection with spirit that sustain a walking practice.

In addition to creating a pattern of walking almost daily, you've been accumulating an assortment of focusing techniques that promote healing and renewal. So far, you've followed weekly walk guidelines as you practice new skills. Now it's time for you to design your own walks. This section provides a summary of focusing techniques from the past seven weeks, and gives you a format to use in outlining your own ongoing walking program.

The techniques are grouped to give you a starting place. Use these lists as a kind of mix-and-match list of possibilities for every walk. Some of the focusing techniques are playful, some prayerful. All of them increase mindfulness, stress release, and connection with self. Let them help you sustain a healthy walking habit and deepen your appreciation for life.

If you decide you prefer the ease of a set walk guideline, go back to Week One and start the Walking Well program over, extending the times of your walks to acknowledge your increased strength and endurance. Repetition will stabilize your exercise routine and increase your familiarity with the focusing tools.

The Basics

These basic focusing techniques form the foundation for many of the "inner walking" tools you've been using in this program. In parentheses is the week where you'll find a more complete description of each exercise.

- *Breathe In, Breathe Out (Week One).* Make breathing a mindful exercise and increase stress release by mentally saying *In* as you inhale and *Out* as you exhale.

- *Put Your Foot Down (Week One).* Get present in your body with full attention to each footstep. Feel the support beneath your feet. Imagine your foot as a rocker, rolling smoothly from heel to toe.

- *Four-Step: In-2-3-4 Cadence (Week One).* Stop mental chatter by counting footsteps. *One-two-three-four, One-two-three-four.*

- *Three-Step: In-2-3 Cadence (Week Three).* Increase focus by using an odd-number count for footsteps. *One-two-three, One two-three,* or *Left-two-three, Right-two-three.*

- *Say Thank You (Week One).* End your walks with a warm heart. Say thank you to your body and to the many things you value in nature and in your life.

The Variations

To keep your focus fresh, you need variety. A change of pace or mental focus can get you back on course when your thoughts veer off to stir up stress. Simply shifting from a four-step rhythm to a three-step pace changes breathing and awareness. When you find processes that work especially well for you, make them a regular part of the rotation in your daily walks. If you want an aerobic segment, include one of the interval workouts a couple times a week.

BREATH FOCUS

- *Clear the Air (Week Two).* Refuel your cells and your spirit. Imagine inhaling fresh energy. Exhale carbon dioxide, tension, anything you'd like to release.

- *Yin-Yang Breath: Earth and Sky (Week Two).* Balance yin and yang as you breathe. Inhale the earth's yin energy of receptivity. Exhale, and feel sky's yang energy of action flow down through your head.

- *Love In, Fear Out (Week Four).* Open your heart to love as you inhale and exhale. Try these variations:

Three-step cadence: *Love comes in, Fear goes out.*
Four-step cadence: *Love comes to me, Fear goes from me.*

- **Compassionate Heart (Week Seven).** Fill your heart with loving kindness. Inhale love through your feet. Exhale and feel love flow from the crown of your head to wash over your body. Inhale, and then exhale love to an individual. Finally, inhale and extend love to your community.

WORDS AND SELF-TALK

- **Four-Step: In-2-3-4 Cadence (Week Two).** Turn the four-step into a cadence that brings words, steps, and breath together. As you count, inhale four steps, exhale four steps.

- **Three-Step: In-2-3 Cadence (Week Three).** Balance brain and body with a three-step cadence of breath, steps, and words: *In-two-three, Out-two-three.* Or focus on your feet: *Left-two-three, Right-two-three.*

- **Mental Marinade: Here/Strong (Week Three).** Take control of self-talk with a three-step cadence that supports breathing and self-appreciation: *I am here, I am strong.* Inhale three words; exhale three words.

- **Change the Marinade (Week Three).** Stir up your own mental marinade that supports and strengthens you with a cadence of words, breath, and steps. For example:
    Three-step marinade: *I am here, I am calm. I am here, I am safe.*
    Four-step marinade: *I am walk-ing, I am heal-ing. I am here and, I am mov-ing.*

I'VE GOT RHYTHM

- *Waltz Walking (Week Five).* Let a song turn your walk into a waltz by adding a mental melody to the three-step cadence. Set the *In-two-three, Out-two-three* pattern to the "Blue Danube," "Greensleeves," or "My Favorite Things."

- *Four-Step Cadence, Sousa Style (Week Five).* Music lightens your steps in a four-step cadence when you find the beat of a march or four-beat song. "Yankee Doodle Dandy" or "Every Time I Feel the Spirit" are energetic starters.

- *Every Little Cell (Week Five).* Sing to yourself as you walk and affirm that your body is healing with each step with a variation on "Shortnin' Bread." See page 112 for a version I like.

POSTURE AND VISUAL IMAGERY

- *Strong and Smooth Image (Week Four).* Imagine your foot as a rocker to add visual imagery to stride and posture. Three-step cadence: *I am strong, I am smooth.*

- *Smooth and Tall Image (Week Four).* Get a lift from imagination with smooth rocker feet and an overhead cable. Three-step cadence: *I am smooth, I am tall.*

- *Bungee Cord (Week Four).* Set your sights on your goal with an imaginary bungee cord. Let it pull you forward to the next tree or streetlight.

- *Guiding Light (Week Six).* Let light be your goal as you walk. Make a game of spotting the gleam that bounces off a passing car or the patch of sun that lights a picket fence.

HEART AND SENSES

- *Sensory Scan (Week Six).* Get present, wherever you are, by using your senses to connect with the world as you walk. Focus on sight, sound, smell, and feeling, giving each sense full attention for a few minutes.

- *Four-Count Sensory Scan (Week Six).* Try a four-step variation by creating a cadence of words, breath, and steps. Repeat mentally, *I am here and, I am see-ing.* After a few minutes, switch focus: *I am here and, I am hear-ing,* and so on.

- *Aerobic Heart Intervals (Week Seven).* Build cardio fitness with cycles of speed walking followed by recovery. Accelerate for fifty steps, then slow to a normal pace for fifty steps. Repeat the cycle three or four times.

- *Bungee Cord Intervals (Week Seven).* For an aerobic variation on bungee cord imagery, attach your imaginary bungee to a goal ahead of you. Accelerate pace until you reach the end of the bungee cord. Recover for an equal distance and then repeat.

EMERGENCY STEPS

- *High Five.* When schedules fall apart, a five-minute oxygen infusion helps put you back together. Get a boost in energy that can last up to two hours with a brisk five-minute walk.

Put It Together

To start your thinking about combinations of techniques that you can assemble in your walks, take a look at these suggestions. Then fill out your own walk plan for Week Eight below. Design two walks so you have variety. Fill in your time goals for each of the walk plans. Use this format in the weeks ahead as you establish a walking practice that sustains health and well-being.

Example Walk 1

1. Clear the Air
2. Waltz Walking: Three-Step
3. Bungee Cord
4. Say Thank You

Example Walk 2

1. Four-Count Sensory Scan: See, Hear, Smell, Feel
2. Three-Step: In-2-3 Cadence
3. Change the Marinade: Three- or Four-Step
4. Say Thank You

Example Walk 3

1. Breathe In, Breathe Out
2. Four-Step: In-2-3-4 Cadence
3. Aerobic Heart Intervals
4. Every Little Cell
5. Say Thank You

Example Walk 4

1. Put Your Foot Down
2. Smooth and Tall Image: Three-Step
3. Yin-Yang Breath: Earth and Sky
4. Say Thank You

Week Eight Goals Overview

Walk Level	Walk Time Goal	Silent Segment Time Goal
Stepping Out	Walk 6 days 20–24 min. a day	10 min. silent
Mid-Stride	Walk 6 days 30 min. a day	15–20 min. silent
Strong and Steady	Walk 6 days 30 min. 4 days 45 min. 2 days	20–30 min. silent

Week Eight Daily Walk Guidelines

Your Level	Focusing Techniques	Time Goal
Walk 1 Time: Days:	1. 2. 3. 4. 5.	
Walk 2 Time: Days:	1. 2. 3. 4. 5.	

Log In and Log On

Use the Week Eight log to record your experiences this week as you plan your own walks. Do you have some favorite focusing techniques already? As you make notes, don't forget to thank yourself and others who have supported your commitment to this healing journey. Give thanks for your willingness to experiment with new ways of thinking and moving. You've been taking significant steps to bring stability and renewal into your life.

As you continue to walk, make the log an ongoing part of your walking practice. The information you collect guides you in making changes to strengthen your commitment to healing and personal well-being. Make a note of mood as well as length of walks. Jot down something special you saw or experienced on this walk. A miracle? A smile? Logs provide motivation as well as a record of your success and your patterns of self-sabotage.

Make copies of the log in the appendix to use in coming weeks, or log on to www.walksthatheal.com for a log you can print out. If you'd like to use the Internet for log-keeping, a search for walking logs will produce a number of sites that help you track distance, time, and frequency of your walks. The best method is the one that works for you.

Moving On

*Facing the Future,
One Step at a Time*

*I*n the warm flush of spring, when nurseries bloom with the promise of summer and gardeners start making plant lists, the facilitator of my cancer support group issued a challenge. She suggested that each participant select a flower to tend and nurture through this growing season. We should designate one specific plant, she insisted, not simply commit to fill the patio planters. Choose something that has special appeal or meaning. Then care for it, as we would like to be cared for ourselves, she advised.

One year out of treatment, I met weekly with this group of survivors, each of us working to find the new "normal" of lives changed by a brush with mortality. Even before the facilitator completed her proposal, I could see the three stark stems of the rose bush I planted the past weekend behind the house. I tried to push the image away. The rose made me nervous. Too vulnerable to insects and disease. Too needy and high risk.

I grew up behind a border of roses that ringed my childhood home. They'd left barbed memories of fish fertilizers, aphid sprays, and fastidious prunings. For years, I'd assiduously avoided these high-maintenance garden divas. The bare-root climbing rose I dug into the soil a few days earlier was the first I'd ever planted. The blank canvas of a new fence had made me bold. Joseph's Coat, a rambling red and gold climber, would splash the boards with color, brightening the kitchen window view. Simply planting my first rose felt risky enough. Adopting a rose pushed my daring. But the rose had its thorns in me. I couldn't shake the image loose.

At home, I stood before the leafless stalks protruding from the ground and surrendered. "Josefina" would be my responsibility and my mirror for this assignment. Together we'd stretch and survive.

My vision reaches again into the future and dares to imagine a landscape that I'll be here to watch, I wrote in my journal at that time. *It is a landscape that now includes a closer proximity to the risks that accompany life's course. Risks that can't be ignored. And here I am, caught on the thorns of a tenacious metaphor that reminds me that I, too, have become a high-maintenance plant. Brambly and ambitious. Vulnerable to disease. In spite of resounding evidence of my body's restored health and vigor, vulnerability shadows me each time I fill my pillbox of medicines and supplements. Life is now more precious, and more precarious.*

Both Josefina and I have weathered health risks and setbacks. Nothing as sobering as the cancer that brought us together eight years ago, but we've both demanded interventions for infections and accidents. High maintenance has become the new normal in my life.

As you move on, traveling a path of personal healing and recovery, you may recognize the need for high maintenance, too. Give yourself opportunities to do the things that heal you—walking, journaling, singing, working, laughing with family and friends. Healing is an incremental process. Take it one step at a time. Each time you move forward, your steps plant an affirmation of your intention to survive. A walk becomes more than a physical gesture; it is a demonstration of commitment, courage, and control. The motivation rises from within.

Commitment and control stand out as defining character traits of resiliency and survival. In a six-year study of 400 career employees who lost jobs in corporate downsizing, nearly two-thirds experienced significant declines in health, including severe stress, heart attacks, depression, and obesity. Those who avoided mental and physical illness demonstrated commitment by staying involved with the events of life rather than withdrawing. They maintained control where they could by finding ways to influence events rather than lapse into helplessness.[1]

You're exhibiting both commitment and control by implementing a walking practice based on the Walking Well guidelines. Commitment has enabled you make time for daily walks that set recovery and healing in motion. Control allows you to shift focus from what has been lost to what is still possible. Both commitment and control lend support each time you summon cognitive override, the mental agility that redirects worries and encourages stress release. It's commitment and control that pull you through when the going is slow and the outcome uncertain.

I bristle at the simplistic suggestion that reduces survival to a cliché: "When life gives you lemons, make lemonade." The breezy formula fails to mention just how much effort it takes to produce this transformation. You can't just set the lemons on a ledge and stare at them. What you'll get is a dry interior and a brittle shell. Instead, you have to take control and squeeze the lemons; extract as much juice as you can. Then discard the pits and bitter peel. Finally, you must sweeten the mix to make it palatable. But where do you turn for the sweetener that blunts the sharp bite of a lemon? Friendship? Love? Family? Faith? Goals? Gratitude? Purpose? Somehow, it's up to you to refine the raw materials of life and extract a buffering ingredient.

Once you acknowledge all the steps involved, the lemons-to-lemonade cliché becomes an apt metaphor for survivorship, for moving on, and making something satisfying out of a trying situation. Perhaps the recipe begins with standing up and getting back on your feet. And I suspect that gratitude is an essential element of the sweetener that completes the transformation.

Gratitude, like walking, is a practice of balance. Hard times narrow our vision to the crisis at hand, shrinking our focus to fear and loss. Gratitude enables us to open the lens through which we see our world. We glimpse blessings as well as burdens. You need not deny or discount the pain of hard times. But your view must expand to include what else is true in your body and your life.

By walking with awareness, you've been expanding vistas both external and internal. By ending your walks with gratitude, you're acknowledging what's right, as well as what's wrong.

What You See Is What You Get

Whether your journey of healing leads you over city sidewalks or rural trails, it's inevitable that sooner or later your steps will lead to a deposit of something unpleasant at your feet. If you're aware and mindful, you'll sidestep it, avoiding a direct encounter with the residue left by another traveler on your path. It's like the once popular bumper sticker proclaimed, in language bold and explicit: "Shit happens."

In teaching walking workshops, I've encountered opportunities to contemplate that expression on trails across the United States. Some have been beautiful and rural, some as common as a parking lot. Participants in these walks confront it, too. Frequently I introduce the Sensory Scan focusing technique that you have used to enhance awareness of your surroundings. By giving attention to what can be seen, heard, smelled, or felt, walkers get present—in the moment and in the setting.

"What did you notice?" I ask when we pause after a few minutes of Sensory Scan walking. "What did your senses reveal?"

"The sound of the breeze rustling in the trees," someone may say. "The smell of sage in the desert. The warmth of the sunshine. A bird sitting on the lamppost. The sound of gravel underfoot."

Eventually, the comments shift. Someone clears a throat and cautiously mentions the "droppings" on the path. "Did you step in it?" I ask. With the laughter comes awareness. We all encounter unpleasantness on life's path, but maybe, if you are being mindful, you don't have to carry it home.

The metaphor expanded a few years ago when I followed a tai chi master on a silent mindfulness hike in the desert bluffs of Southern California. As we set out, I settled into a three-count rhythm to steady my mind and calm my impatience with the slow, deliberate pace. The route led up a gentle mountain trail and wound down to a shaded labyrinth where we followed ancient circuits into the center and back. All along the mountain trail, dark droppings affirmed the popularity of this path with the local coyote population. As I mulled the presence of this visual blight, a smile began to form. Those wily coyotes had deposited a lesson at my feet: What lay on the trail was simply the waste product of substances that once provided food and fuel. Stripped of useful nutrients, the coyotes discarded the waste and left it behind. The metaphor followed me into the labyrinth, where my footsteps gradually guided me to a subtle recognition of the similarities of shape in the coils of the sacred labyrinth and those of a human digestive tract.

"Leave it on the trail!" my mind shouted in delight as the insight settled into my cells. "Use it and then let it go."

On any path, an encounter with scat at my feet reminds me to discard what no longer sustains and nourishes me. This is not an excuse for irresponsible pet owners who ignore sanitation policies. But rather than dwell on outrage or indignation, it offers me an alternative perspective on a natural phenomenon. On the mountain trails I love to travel, the droppings affirm the rhythms of life, of taking in and letting go.

Hanging on is a hindrance to moving on. It's true that anger, fear, bitterness, and sorrow are vital and useful at times. Caution, stubbornness, persistence, and pain serve a purpose, too. Take what you need from life's emotions and experiences. Use them to motivate action, or to protect you from overreaction. Let them guide you in knowing what is important. Then know when it's time to walk away. Only you can decide when the nutrient value of an emotion or experience is depleted. Walking helps.

The metaphors of movement keep you grounded and moving forward. The cycle of breath reminds you to open up to fresh air and new perspectives, and then release the spent residue. The walks that have brought you to this point become the foundation for the walks ahead, both physical and spiritual. The best walks deliver more than exercise; they lead to connection with spirit.

A Walk before the Storm

Architect Bob Barr loves to walk along the coastal edge of the Isle of Iona. He turns left as he disembarks from the ferry that delivers travelers to the tiny island off the coast of Scotland. Not right, to the gray stone structures of the village. Not toward the lofty arches of the abbey or the shrine of St. Columba, revered as a Christian pilgrimage site. Instead, he heads south on a country road, past a solitary white cottage sparkling in the sunlight. His wife walks at his side. They pause to marvel at the cottage garden, a profusion of color, from front gate to front door. Bright blossoms blaze with welcoming warmth.

Beyond the house, they pass the three-hole golf course where a lone player walks the fairway with no bag, just two clubs carried casually in hand. On down the road, twenty minutes or so, the route rises to overlook the sea, intensely blue in the light of day. Waves crash against the rocky coastline, sending foamy spray fifteen feet into the air. The view, he says, takes your breath away.

It also banishes stress.

Bob's enchantment with the island began on a rare sunny day when he and his wife set out on these rural roadways with the intention of walking a full circuit around the small island where tourist cars and buses are banned. They had come to Iona with a group of Presbyterian travelers who were visiting sacred sites in Scotland. But they'd wearied of village teashops and hushed cloisters. After several days of wet, dreary weather, a bright break in the skies overhead sealed their decision to turn their steps toward a country road, and skip the village. They were eager for the movement and quiet meditation of a rural saunter. A reasonably fit person, they'd been assured, could walk the island circuit in two hours, plenty of time to get back for the scheduled ferry departure for the mainland. They'd been walking thirty or forty minutes when they reached the western outcroppings of the island, with ocean and cliffs before them. They gasped in wonder at the sun-splashed sea, and then they looked at one another. They sat down on the grass in silence, enraptured by the scene. With few vehicles on the island, the only sounds they heard were nature's sounds: the waves, the birds, the rustle of wind in the heathers.

"We just sat, being quiet, entranced with ocean waves, and the sounds of the water," he recalls.[2] "We sat long enough that we knew we couldn't make the full circuit around the island. We'd have to return the way we came. But it was emotionally so pleasing. Really, it felt like a spiritual experience, with the earth and with God."

Reverend George MacLeod, founder of a twentieth-century spiritual community on the island, would have nodded in agreement. MacLeod describes Iona as "a thin place," where earth and heaven almost touch. When the Barrs walked away from that thin place and returned to their home in the United States, they knew they had experienced something significant on Iona. They didn't yet know how often they would repeat that walk, as a path of peace in times of overwork, illness, and stress. They didn't know that twelve years later it would lead them through a medical crisis that put Bob's life in danger.

As a managing partner in an international architecture firm based in Washington, D.C., Bob is no stranger to stress and tension. Deadlines, budgets, and client expectations bring pressure to every project. When he returned from Iona, he discovered that he could retreat from the stress by returning to the island mentally, in a bedtime meditation. At night, he'd lie in bed and picture the road that led past the white house and beyond the golf greens. He'd walk along the coastal bluff and listen for the crash of waves, letting the sound of wind and water lull him into sleep.

A few years later, when a stroke shook his hold on life, he prepared for triple bypass surgery by traveling the soothing path once again, out to the island's western tip. In the pre-surgery holding area, his wife stood beside a hospital gurney and held his hand. Together they talked the walk. "Remember when we first glimpsed the white house? The thatched roof? Those amazing flowers? So many flowers. Remember that little golf course, and the golfer with two clubs?" Step by step they moved through the walk, noting details of landscape, color, and sound, until they sat together on the grass, watching clouds and cliffs and the play of sunlight on the sea. "Mentally, I kept going over that walk and the beauty of it," he recalls. "With the memory of the flowers and the house and the grass and the hills, I felt very calm. And when I finished the mental walk, I felt ready for surgery."

Bob emerged from a medical crisis with renewed commitment to changes in stress management, diet, and lifestyle. Walking took on fresh importance. He walks often with his wife, and he also walks alone. When a flight is delayed or a work deadline moved up, he retreats to the coastline of Iona and travels the familiar path in his mind. When sleep evades him, he blocks words of worry by listening to the roar of waves.

"Walking is precious," he says. "You can do the same path every day and see something different."

Facing the Future

You need not journey to the Isle of Iona or walk miles on ancient paths to reach that thin place where earth and heaven almost touch. Move the body and you move the spirit, no matter where you walk. Move the body and healing emerges in the alchemy of breath and movement that restores wholeness and soothes the soul. The mindfulness skills you've brought to your walks on this eight-week program help get you there.

Focus on breath, and you focus on spirit, the source of life and inspiration. A focus on words shapes a prayer that turns awareness to intention and gratitude. The steps you've taken to bring body and mind together recognize that healing isn't simply a physical process, but also an emotional, spiritual, and mental journey—a journey of survival.

With a walking practice that keeps you moving forward, you've set in motion the rhythms of recovery. As you continue, stepping into the future, take with you the practices that have enhanced stress release, attitude, or posture. Take the schedule of daily walks you've established. Make a list of the focusing techniques that work best for you and let go of those that don't. Let go of judgments about how far or how often you walked. Say thank you regularly. Sustain the practice with commitment and compassion.

The patterns that emerge from your steps infuse each day with healing. Out of healing comes purpose—a way to go forward in life motivated by intention rather than by fear.

SIDE STEPS: *Walking and Aging*

Aging may not be an illness, but it can certainly set off a sequence of traumas. From the first wrinkles and gray hairs to the nagging fears of memory loss, the changes that accompany the passage of time often feel very painful. Exercise, healthy food, and a good attitude go a long way in postponing or preventing many of the disabilities and diseases we associate with aging.

It's true that staying fit is pretty much a case of use it or lose it. But fitness isn't necessarily lost and gone forever. Even if you've let exercise slide, a number of studies offer reassurance that it's never too late to increase life expectancy and health with exercise. From physical mobility to mental agility, exercise may be the closest thing to a fountain of youth that we've found.

WALK MORE, LIVE MORE

A daily walk of two miles adds up to a longer life, according to a twelve-year study, which showed that death rates dropped 19 percent for each mile a person consistently walked daily. The research, based on the Honolulu Heart Program, followed 707 nonsmoking, able-bodied men age sixty-one to eighty-one. In all, 208 of the men died in the twelve-year study period, but the amount of walking appeared significant for those who survived. For people who walked two miles a day, odds of survival were twice as high as for those who walked infrequently.[3]

LATE STARTERS FINISH STRONG

A Swedish study of 2,205 nonexercisers who entered fitness programs at age fifty confirmed that any time is a good time to start exercising. Follow-up evaluations of participants at ages seventy, seventy-seven, and eighty-two showed that men who did the most exercise lived an average of 2.3 years longer, and men who did moderate exercise lived 1.1 years longer than men who reported the lowest levels.[4]

BUFF UP YOUR BRAIN

The Alzheimer's Association predicts that ten million baby boomers will develop Alzheimer's disease in the United States. The statistics are frightening, but studies repeatedly point to exercise as a defense against this condition. "Regular exercise is probably the best means we have of preventing Alzheimer's disease today, better than medication, better than intellectual activity, better than supplements and diets," says Dr. Ronald Peterson, director of the Alzheimer's Research Center at the Mayo Clinic. Researchers recommend exercise that raises your heart rate for thirty minutes several times a week, increasing blood flow and oxygen to the brain.[5]

A healthy diet combined with regular physical activity boosted the odds of avoiding Alzheimer's disease by 59 percent for a group of New Yorkers aged seventy and over. The study by Columbia University assessed diet and physical activity levels of almost 2,000 participants for five years. A healthy diet and exercise each independently protect against Alzheimer's, but this study showed that when the two are combined, the benefits are even greater.[6]

Vascular dementia, the second most common form of cognitive impairment associated with aging, can also be lessened with a regular program of moderate exercise. Walking was associated with a 73 percent reduction in vascular dementia in a study that analyzed exercise and lifestyle of men and women aged sixty-five and older.[7] Vascular dementia results from chronic reduced blood flow in the brain and is characterized by a slow, progressive loss of memory and other cognitive functions.

IT'S THE THOUGHT THAT COUNTS

A positive attitude helped seniors walk faster and with better posture in a study at Boston's Beth Israel Deaconess Hospital. Participants in the study walked the length of a football field as researchers measured walking speed and form. Then walkers viewed a computer game embedded with subliminal messages. Half the walkers received words like *accomplished, wise,* and *astute* that convey an upbeat view of aging. Half received negative words like *senile, dependent,* and *diseased.* On a second walk, the participants who received positive mental suggestions walked faster and with improved form. Performance in the negative group was unchanged, perhaps because the subliminal messages merely echoed stereotypes we already hold about age.[8]

Acknowledgments

My deep gratitude to all who have supported my healing, my explorations, and my evolving appreciation for walking as a vehicle of fitness, wholeness, joy, and healing. So many teachers and companions have guided and shaped this book.

First, I acknowledge the generous, trusting people who agreed to share their personal stories of hard times and of healing steps with the readers of *Healing Walks for Hard Times*. You have enriched this project with life experiences that reveal the profound rewards of healing walks. To the researchers and writers who have deepened my understanding of walking, healing, and moving on, I give thanks for your contributions to this project.

To Trish Martin, fitness director at the Golden Door Resort, I give thanks for encouraging and mentoring my steps from writer to speaker. And, to the trusting walkers who joined me for meadow walks at the Door, I give thanks for enthusiasm and patience as I learned to share my zeal for walking.

To Susan Leigh, RN, and Robert Brooks, MD, I give thanks for the vision and commitment that have fueled Life Beyond Cancer Retreats at Miraval, and for inviting me into the family of survivors and thrivers assembled by this event. To James Lasker, MD, whose support for healing walks has been steady and generous, I give great thanks. A Lasker Foundation writing grant supported development of this book.

To Kathy LaTour and the staff of *Cure* magazine and seminars, I give thanks for encouragement, and for the leadership that produced a national network of healing opportunities for people facing the challenges of cancer. To Willamette Valley Cancer Institute and Research Center in Eugene, Oregon, I give thanks for compassionate guidance in my own healing journey, and for the opportunity to try out a parking lot version of the Walking Well program for patients and families.

To members of my writing group, I offer humble appreciation for patience, honesty, and unflagging faith: Elizabeth Lyon, Mabel Armstrong, Geraldine Moreno Black, Barbara Corrado Pope, and Faris Cassell. Also, to my agent, Catherine Fowler of the Redwood Agency.

To every person who has joined me for a walk, who has stopped to tell me how walking has enriched their lives, who has been willing to experiment with bringing mind-body focus to their walks, I give thanks. You motivate and inspire me. To the many spiritual and physical mentors who have guided my steps and accompanied my journey, I offer reverent appreciation.

And to Dean, my favorite walking companion, love and gratitude always.

Appendix

Weekly Walking Logs

Walking Well Sample Log

Date: _May 15–22_ **Goal or desired outcome this week:** _Connection with nature_

Walk Days	Walk Time		Silent Segment	Health and Fitness Notes	Nature Notes, Comments, Appreciation
Sun.	Goal	20 min.	10 min.	No pain in knee! Moderate energy	Crisp morning, cool, fresh air. Saw two housefinches on feeder. Love my new shoes and feeling ground under my feet.
	Done	23 min.	23 min.		
Tues.	Goal	20 min.	15 min.	Challeng-ing to breathe in and out nose	Vibrant sunset this evening. New mari-golds planted at corner house. Fo-cused on counting steps. Helpful.
	Done	25 min.	10 min.		
Wed.	Goal	20 min.	10 min.	Tired to-day. Up late last night. Mood bet-ter after walk.	Windy, smell of mown grass in air. Cool breeze helped wake me up! Count-ing steps clears head.
	Done	15 min.	10 min.		
Thur.	Goal	25 min.	15 min.		
	Done				
Fri.	Goal	25 min.			
	Done				
Sat.	Goal	20 min.			
	Done				

Walking Well—Week One: A Healthy Step

Date: _____ ***Goal or desired outcome this week:*** _____

Walk Days	Walk Time		Silent Segment	Health and Fitness Notes	Nature Notes, Comments, Appreciation
	Goal				
	Done				
	Goal				
	Done				
	Goal				
	Done				
	Goal				
	Done				
	Goal				
	Done				
	Goal				
	Done				

Walking Well—Week Two: A Healthy Spirit

Date: _____ Goal or desired outcome this week: _____

Walk Days	Walk Time		Silent Segment	Health and Fitness Notes	Nature Notes, Comments, Appreciation
	Goal				
	Done				
	Goal				
	Done				
	Goal				
	Done				
	Goal				
	Done				
	Goal				
	Done				
	Goal				
	Done				

Walking Well—Week Three: A Healthy Mind

Date: _____ ***Goal or desired outcome this week:*** _____

Walk Days	Walk Time		Silent Segment	Health and Fitness Notes	Nature Notes, Comments, Appreciation
	Goal				
	Done				
	Goal				
	Done				
	Goal				
	Done				
	Goal				
	Done				
	Goal				
	Done				
	Goal				
	Done				

Walking Well—Week Four: A Healthy Self-Image

Date: _____ *Goal or desired outcome this week:* _____

Walk Days	Walk Time		Silent Segment	Health and Fitness Notes	Nature Notes, Comments, Appreciation
	Goal				
	Done				
	Goal				
	Done				
	Goal				
	Done				
	Goal				
	Done				
	Goal				
	Done				
	Goal				
	Done				

Walking Well—Week Five: A Healthy Rhythm

Date: _____ *Goal or desired outcome this week:* _____

Walk Days	Walk Time		Silent Segment	Health and Fitness Notes	Nature Notes, Comments, Appreciation
	Goal				
	Done				
	Goal				
	Done				
	Goal				
	Done				
	Goal				
	Done				
	Goal				
	Done				
	Goal				
	Done				

Walking Well—Week Six: A Healthy Attitude

Date: _____ *Goal or desired outcome this week:* _____

Walk Days	Walk Time		Silent Segment	Health and Fitness Notes	Nature Notes, Comments, Appreciation
	Goal				
	Done				
	Goal				
	Done				
	Goal				
	Done				
	Goal				
	Done				
	Goal				
	Done				
	Goal				
	Done				

Walking Well—Week Seven: A Healthy Heart

Date: _____ *Goal or desired outcome this week:* _____

Walk Days	Walk Time		Silent Segment	Health and Fitness Notes	Nature Notes, Comments, Appreciation
	Goal				
	Done				
	Goal				
	Done				
	Goal				
	Done				
	Goal				
	Done				
	Goal				
	Done				
	Goal				
	Done				

Walking Well—Week Eight: A Healthy Habit

Date: _____ *Goal or desired outcome this week:* _____

Walk Days	Walk Time		Silent Segment	Health and Fitness Notes	Nature Notes, Comments, Appreciation
	Goal				
	Done				
	Goal				
	Done				
	Goal				
	Done				
	Goal				
	Done				
	Goal				
	Done				
	Goal				
	Done				

Moving On

Date: _____ *Goal or desired outcome this week:* _____

Walk Days	Walk Time		Silent Segment	Health and Fitness Notes	Nature Notes, Comments, Appreciation
	Goal				
	Done				
	Goal				
	Done				
	Goal				
	Done				
	Goal				
	Done				
	Goal				
	Done				
	Goal				
	Done				

Notes

Starting Out

1. Thich Nhat Hanh, *Present Moment, Wonderful Moment* (Berkeley, Calif.: Parallax Press, 1990), 3.

Week One

1. Nola Woodbury, interview by author, March 17, 1999.
2. Al Siebert, *The Resiliency Advantage* (San Francisco: Berrett-Koehler Publishers, 2005), 32.
3. Herbert Benson, with William Proctor, *Beyond the Relaxation Response* (New York: Times Books, 1984), 138.
4. Rory Stewart, *The Places in Between* (Orlando: Harcourt Books, 2006), 76.
5. Dan Baker and Cameron Stauth, *What Happy People Know: How the New Science of Happiness Can Change Your Life for the Better* (New York: St. Martin's, 2003), 82.
6. Robert A. Emmons and Michael McCullough, "Highlights from the research project on gratitude and thankfulness," http://psychology .ucdavis.edu/labs/emmons/ (accessed June 14, 2008).
7. Suzanne Segerstrom, PhD, and Gregory Miller, PhD, "Psychological stress and the human immune system: A meta-analytic study of 30 years of inquiry," *Psychological Bulletin* 130 (2004): 4.
8. Medline Plus, "Medical encyclopedia: Exercise and immunity," www.nlm.nih.gov/medlineplus/ency/article/007165.htm (accessed August 23, 2009).
9. David C. Nieman, "Does exercise alter immune function and respiratory infections?" *Research Digest,* President's Council on Physical Fitness and Sports (June 2001): 1.
10. "University of Wisconsin study reports sustained changes in brain

and immune function after meditation," *ScienceDaily* (February 4, 2003), www.sciencedaily.com/releases/2003/02/030204074125.htm (accessed March 19, 2008).

11. Benson with Proctor, *Beyond the Relaxation Response,* 138.

12. Ibid., 138.

Week Two

1. Robert E. Thayer, telephone interview by author, Nov. 6, 2008.

2. Stephen Gaudet, telephone interview by author, May 5, 2009; e-mail interview with author, May 4, 2009.

3. Thayer, telephone interview by author, Nov. 6, 2008.

4. Robert E. Thayer, *The Origin of Everyday Moods: Managing Energy, Tension, and Stress* (New York: Oxford University Press, 1996), 29. Cites: J. K. Dixon, J. P. Dixon, and M. Hickey, "Energy as a central factor in the self-assessment of health," *Advances in Nursing Science* 15 (1993): 1–12.

5. Timothy W. Puetz, Patrick J. O'Connor, and Rod K. Dishman, "Effects of exercise on feelings of energy and fatigue: A quantitative synthesis," *Psychological Bulletin* 132, no. 6 (Nov. 2006): 866–876.

Week Three

1. Terry Gray, telephone interview by author, July 26, 2006.

2. Martin E. P. Seligman, *Authentic Happiness* (New York: Free Press, 2002), 31–39.

3. Jacqueline Meehan, telephone interview by author, May 9, 2009.

4. Herbert Benson, with Marg Stark, *Timeless Healing: The Power and Biology of Belief* (New York: Scribner, 1996), 272.

5. Nick Symmonds, "Training diary," *The Register-Guard* (Eugene, Ore.), June 5, 2008, E6.

6. Jeffrey M. Hausdorff, Becca R. Levy, and Jeanne Y. Wei, "The power of ageism on physical function of older persons: Reversibility of age-related gait changes," *Journal of the American Geriatrics Society* 47, no. 11 (Nov. 1999): 1346–1349.

7. John Ratey, "Working out your issues," *Washington Post,* June 14, 2005, F1.

8. Duke University Medical Center, "Effect of exercise on reducing major depression appears to be long-lasting," September 21, 2000, www.charitywire.com/charity280/04727.html (accessed August 23, 2009).

9. Holisticonline.com, "Depression and exercise," http://holisticonline.com/Remedies/Depression/dep_exercise.htm (accessed April 12, 2009).

10. Robert E. Thayer, *Calm Energy: How People Regulate Mood with Food and Exercise* (New York, Oxford University Press, 2001), 34.

Week Four

1. Tammey Burns, telephone interview by author, June 29, 2009.
2. Colleen Young, telephone interview by author, June 26, 2009.
3. Robert Dinsmoor, "Strength training after sixty," *Harvard Health Letter* 18, no. 9 (July 1993), 6–8.
4. Stephen Kiesling and E. C. Frederick, *Walk On: A Tool Kit for Building Your Own Walking Fitness Program* (Emmaus, Penn.: Rodale Press, 1986), 70.
5. Dinsmoor, "Strength training after sixty."

Week Five

1. Norman Nicholson, ed., *The Lake District: An Anthology* (London: Penguin Books, 1978), 143.
2. Andrew Weil, *Spontaneous Healing* (New York: Knopf, 1995), 188.
3. Peggy Peck, "Daily doses of Bach and breathing lower blood pressure," *MedPage Today,* May 23, 2008. Cites: Pietro A. Modesti and Gianfranco Parati, "Daily sessions of music can reduce 24-hour ambulatory blood pressure in mild hypertension," Presentation, American Society of Hypertension, New Orleans, 2008, www.medpagetoday.com/MeetingCoverage/ASH/9597 (accessed June 28, 2009).
4. Eknath Easwaran, *Meditation: An Eight-Point Program* (Petaluma, Calif.: Nilgiri Press, 1978), 39.
5. The Holy Bible, Proverbs 23:7.
6. Susan Bartlett, "Role of exercise in the management of arthritis," Physiological Benefits, www.hopkins-arthritis.org/patient-corner/disease-management/exercise.html (accessed June 2, 2009).
7. Chris Bynum, "Finding your rhythm helps you stay in shape," *Times-Picayune,* January 18, 2008.

Week Six

1. Carolee Shaw, telephone interview by author, Dec. 16, 2008.
2. Baker and Stauth, *What Happy People Know,* 37.
3. Viktor E. Frankl, *Man's Search for Meaning* (New York: Simon and Schuster, 1985), 86.
4. Ibid.,135.
5. Dan Baker, telephone interview by author, Nov. 3, 2008.
6. Linda Williamson, e-mail interview by author, Sept. 8–10, 2008.
7. Carl W. Cotman and Nicole C. Berchtold, "Exercise: A behavioral

intervention to enhance brain health and plasticity," *Trends in Neurosciences* 25, no. 6 (June 1, 2002): 295–301, http://dx.doi .org/10.1016/S0166-2236(02)02143-4 (accessed August 3, 2009).

8. K. I. Erickson and A. F. Kramer, "Aerobic exercise effects on cognitive and neural plasticity in older adults," *British Journal of Sports Medicine* 43 (2009): 22–24.

9. Melissa McNamara, "Boosting brain power may be steps away," CBS NEWS, January 17, 2007, www.cbsnews.com/stories/2007/ 01/17/eveningnews/main2368898.shtml?tag=contentMain;content Body (accessed August 24, 2009).

10. Charles H. Hillman, Robert W. Moti, Matthew B. Pontifex, Danielle Posthuma, Janine H. Stubbe, Dorret I. Boomsma, and Eco J.C. deGeus, "Physical activity and cognitive function in a cross-section of younger and older community-dwelling individuals," *Health Psychology* 25, no. 6 (2006): 678–687.

11. Arthur F. Kramer, Sowon Hahn, Neal J. Cohen, Marie T. Banich, Edward McAuley, Catherine R. Harrison, Julie Chason, Eli Vakil, Lunn Bardell, Richard A. Boliau, and Angela Colcomb, "Ageing, fitness and neurocognitive function," *Nature* 400 (1999): 418–419.

12. Jeannine Stein, "Brain function gets a boost from walking," *Los Angeles Times,* Sept. 8, 2008, http://articles.latimes.com/2008/ sep/08/health/he-walking8 (accessed September 13, 2008). Nicola T. Lautenschlager, Kay L. Cox, Leon Flicker, Jonathan K. Foster, Frank M. van Bockxmeer, Jianguo Xiao, Kathryn R. Greenop, and Osvaldo P. Almeida, "Effect of physical activity on cognitive function in older adults at risk for alzheimer disease," *Journal of the American Medical Association (JAMA)* 300, no. 9 (2008): 1027–1037.

13. Dan Baker, *What Happy People Know,* 38.

Week Seven

1. Elvira Crocker, e-mail correspondence with author, May 26, 2009; telephone interview by author, June 3, 2009.

2. Jean Shinoda Bolen, MD, *Close to the Bone: Life-Threatening Illness and the Search for Meaning* (New York: Touchstone, 1996), 18–19.

3. Carlos Castaneda, *The Teachings of Don Juan: A Yaqui Way of Knowledge* (New York: Simon and Schuster, 1968), 160.

4. James Carse, telephone interview by author, July 14, 1997.

5. Timothy S. Church, MD, MPH, PhD; Conrad P. Earnest, PhD; James S. Skinner, PhD; and Steven N. Blair, PED; "Effects of different doses of physical activity on cardio respiratory fitness among sedentary, overweight or obese postmenopausal women with

elevated blood pressure: A randomized controlled trial," *Journal of the American Medical Association (JAMA)* 297, no. 19 (2007): 2081–2091.

6. Warren King, "Heart benefits equally from moderate or strenuous exercise, UW study finds," *Seattle Times,* April 12, 1999, http://community.seattletimes.nwsource.com/archive/?date=19990412&slug=2954728 (accessed April 12, 1999). Cites: Rozenn N. Lemaitre, David S. Siscovick, Trivellore E. Raghunathan, Sheila Weinmann, Patrick Arbogast, and Dan-Yu Lin, "Leisure-time physical activity and the risk of primary cardiac arrest," *Archives of Internal Medicine* 159, no. 7 (1999): 686–690.

7. "New exercise guidelines: In 2009, don't just sit there, do something!" *Tufts University Health and Nutrition Letter,* www.tuftshealthletter.com/ShowArticle.aspx?rowId=671 (accessed July 5, 2009).

8. Simon J. Marshall, Susan S. Levy, Catrine E. Tudor-Locke, Fred W. Kolkhorst, Karen M. Wooten, Ming Ji, Caroline A. Macera, and Barbara E. Ainsworth, "Translating physical activity recommendations into a pedometer-based step goal: 3000 Steps in 30 Minutes," *American Journal of Preventive Medicine* 36, no. 5 (2009): 410–415.

9. Jamie Stengle, "Heart group kicks off fitness campaign," *Associated Press News,* January 9, 2007.

10. "Women with pedometers step up exercise levels," American College of Sports Medicine news release, April 5, 2005, www.acsm.org/AM/Template.cfm?Section=Search&template=/CM/HTMLDisplay.cfm&ContentID=9092 (accessed August 25, 2009).

Week Eight

1. Karen Foto, telephone interview by author, March 30, 2009.

2. Diane Doster, telephone interview by author, July 21, 2009.

3. Robert Thayer, telephone interview by author, Nov. 6, 2008.

4. Carrie Wells, interview by author, July 9, 2005, Washington, D.C.; telephone interview by author, July 20, 2009.

5. Donald Meichenbaum, interview by Victor Yalom, "Cognitive behavioral therapy and trauma," April 2002, www.psychotherapy.net/interview/Donald_Meichenbaum (accessed July 26, 2009).

Moving On

1. American Psychological Association Online, "Turning lemons into lemonade: Hardiness helps people turn stressful circumstances into opportunities," www.psychologymatters.org/hardiness.html# (accessed May 4, 2009).

2. Bob Barr, telephone interview by author, April 22, 2009.

3. Steven Reinberg, "Men who get active in midlife live longer,"

HealthDay News, March 5, 2009, www.healthday.com/printer
.asp?AID=624777 (accessed August 20, 2009).

4. Associated Press, "Walks add years to life, study shows," *New York Times,* January 8, 1998.

5. Angela Lunde, "Preventing Alzheimer's: Exercise still best bet," Alzheimer's Blog, March 25, 2008, www.mayoclinic.com/health/ alzheimers/MY00002 (accessed August 20, 2009).

6. Roni Caryn Rabin, "Prevention: Diet and exercise lower Alzheimer's risk," *New York Times,* August 18, 2009, www.nytimes.com/ 2009/08/18/health/18prev.html (accessed August 22, 2009).

7. "Regular walking may cut vascular dementia risk more than 70%," *Tufts University Health and Nutrition Letter,* March 2008, www.tufts healthletter.com/ShowArticle.aspx?rowld=92, (accessed August 2, 2009).

8. Christiane Northrup, MD, *The Wisdom of Menopause* (New York: Bantam Books, 2001), 326–327. Cites: Jeffrey M. Hausdorff, Becca R. Levy, Jeanne Y Wei, "The power of ageism on physical function of older persons: Reversibility of age-related gait changes," *Journal of the American Geriatrics Society* 47, no. 11 (Nov. 1999): 1346–1349.

Resources

Many books, DVDs, and CDs provide instruction in ways to expand your walking experiences. The following resources provide a good starting place for information about fitness walking.

Andrew Weil and Mark Fenton. *Walking: The Ultimate Exercise for Optimum Health* (Sounds True, 2006). Walking expert Mark Fenton provides a guided walk on the helpful Workout CD included in this two-CD set. An introductory CD by Dr. Weil and Fenton offers inspiration and information about health benefits of walking. On the second CD, Fenton leads walkers through a gentle warm-up and provides a series of walking segments leading up to an aerobic pace.

> *In my opinion, walking is the most healthful form of physical activity, the one that has the greatest capacity to keep the healing system in good working order, and increase the likelihood of spontaneous healing in case of illness.*
> —Andrew Weil, MD, *Spontaneous Healing*

Mark Fenton. *The Complete Guide to Walking, New and Revised: For Health, Weight Loss, and Fitness* (The Lyons Press, 2008). Mark Fenton's practical and personal knowledge of walking has made him a respected authority in the fitness walking world. A former member of the U.S. racewalking team, Fenton has authored a number of walking books and hosts the PBS series *America's Walking*. In *The Complete Guide to Walking*, he provides an excellent all-around guide to posture, stride, walking gear, and schedules. Sections of the book include guidelines on walking for health, for weight loss, for aerobic exercise, and for recreational outings with children.

Carolyn Scott Kortge. *The Spirited Walker: Fitness Walking for Clarity, Balance, and Spiritual Connection* (HarperOne, 1998). Kortge, a former nationally ranked racewalker, introduces an approach to fitness that puts care of the soul on equal footing with care of the body. Easy-to-do visualizations, breathing exercises, and active affirmations transform fitness walks into an active, aerobic meditation. Exercises guide you to use focusing tools the way that athletes do, to strengthen both mind and body. www.spiritedwalker.com.

Walk for a Cause

Community benefit walks provide year-round opportunities to lend your feet to a worthy cause. Many associations host walks to raise funds and awareness for a specific cause or disease. Some offer distance walks of several days. Others provide training programs that support participants in preparing for a walking event.

When you are physically ready, a community walk can be a wonderful way to connect with people who share your interests and concerns. Notices in the local media often announce community events. National organizations maintain websites that point you to walks in your area. For a starting place, here are a few of the most familiar sites. An Internet search will reveal many other groups that encourage you to keep walking.

American Cancer Society Relay for Life:
   www.relayforlife.org/relay

American Heart Association Heart Walk:
   www.startwalkingnow.org/start_heart_walk.jsp

American Diabetes Association StepOut Walk:
   http://stepout.diabetes.org/site/PageServer?pagename=OUT_homepage

Susan G. Komen Race for the Cure:
   ww5.komen.org/findarace.aspx

Arthritis Foundation Arthritis Walk:
   http://lmt.arthritis.org/arthritis-walk/index.php

Leukemia and Lymphoma Society Team in Training
   www.teamintraining.org

About the Author

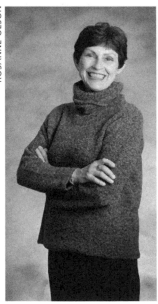

Carolyn Scott Kortge is an award-winning journalist, a former competitive racewalker, a public speaker, and a cancer survivor. She has appeared at nationally renowned resorts and at wellness events from San Diego to Washington, DC. She is also the author of *The Spirited Walker: Fitness Walking for Clarity, Balance, and Spiritual Connection*. Kortge has been featured as an authority on walking for body, mind, and spirit in publications including *Self* magazine, *Family Circle, Woman's Day, Cure, Health,* the *Philadelphia Inquirer, The Oregonian,* and *Bottom Line*. Her writing has appeared in *Newsweek, Hemispheres, GEO, Modern Maturity, The Lutheran,* and numerous newspapers. She's also developed the Walking Well® program, which she has presented at medical centers, wellness events, survivor conferences, and health resorts and spas across the United States.

Index

dogged, 58–60
diabetes, 15
    cases of, 136
    and neuropathy, 170
Doster, Diane, 162, 163, 165
"droppings" on the path, 184–85

emotional balance, 58. *See also*
    balance: mental
emotional heart. *See* heart
    (spiritual/symbolic)
emotions, positive and negative,
    57–58, 60–61
energy
    mood and, 45, 66–67
    walking and, 44–45
equipment, selecting, 8–9
Every Little Cell (rhythmic
    exercise), 112, 176
exercise
    intensity levels of, 146–47
    See also specific topics
exercise logs. *See* Walking Logs
exercises, muscle-strengthening,
    169

fatigue, 45
fear. *See* Love In, Fear Out
feet, 23
    noticing action of, 30–31
    walking and, 168–71
Fifteen-Minute Mood Mender
    (exercise), 67–68
fitness levels, 9–12
focus, rotating, 29
focusing techniques, 29–30,
    172–78
    basic, 173–74
    combinations of, 178
    emergency steps, 177
    heart and senses, 177

posture and visual imagery,
    176–77
rhythm, 176
variations on, 174–75
words and self-talk, 175
See also specific techniques
foot problems and injuries,
    169–71
footsteps. *See* steps
footwork, mindful, 30–32
Foto, Karen, 158–61
Four-Count Sensory Scan
    (focusing technique), 130,
    177
Four-Step: In-2-3-4 Cadence
    (breathing and focusing
    technique), 31–32, 47, 72,
    113, 153, 173, 175
Four-Step Cadence, Sousa Style
    (rhythmic exercise),
    111–12, 176
Frankl, Viktor, 119
fundraising walks, 76–78, 102,
    166–68, 213
future, facing the, 188–89

Gaudet, Stephen, 41–43
germs, spread of, 27
goals. *See* walking goals
gratitude, 24–25, 131, 183–84.
    See also Say Thank You
Gray, Terry, 2, 54–57, 69
grief. *See* death of a loved one
Griest, John, 66
Guiding Light (focusing tech-
    nique), 130, 177

habits
    forming, 161–63
    healthy, 158, 160–61
    practice and, 172

Meehan, Jacqueline, 58–60, 69
Meichenbaum, Donald, 168
memory, 127
mental balance. *See* balance
mental clarity, 16
"mental marinades," 60–61
　creating new, positive, 63–65
　See also Change the Marinade
Mental Marinades: Here/Strong
　(self-talk tool), 71, 153, 175
Mental Marinades: Three- or
　Four-Count Cadence (self-
　talk tool), 131
mental music, 103–7
Mid-Stride—Moderate Level, 11
mindfulness, 17, 21
mindfulness techniques, 29–32.
　See also specific techniques
miracles, 128
mitochondria, 45
moderation, importance of,
　32–33
mood
　energy and, 45, 66–67
　walking and, 65–68
mood-mender walk, 67–68
Mothers Against Drunk Driving
　(MADD), 168
motivation, 161–62, 164–65
movement
　begins with the will to move,
　　xiii
　metaphors of, 184–86
　mindfulness and, 17
muscles, walking and, 86–87
music, 103–7

negativity and negative self-talk,
　60–61. *See also* emotions;
　self-talk
Nelson, Miriam, 146

neuropathy, 170
obesity, cases of, 82–86
"one step at a time," 1, 7, 25,
　38, 182
　chanting and, 37–39, 41, 105
　cognitive override and, 5
osteoarthritis, 107–8, 170
osteoporosis, 15

pace
　aerobic, 150–51
　and heart health, 147–49
path with heart, a, 139–45
pedometer, 147–49
personal stories
　Bob Barr, 186–88
　Carolee Shaw, 116–20
　Carrie Wells, 165–67
　Elvira Valenzuela Crocker,
　　135–37
　Jacqueline Meehan, 58–60,
　　69
　Karen Foto, 158–61
　Linda Williamson, 122–25,
　　130
　Nick Symmonds, 61–62
　Nola Woodbury, 17–19
　Stephen Gaudet, 41–43
　"Suzanne," 102–3
　Tammey Burns, 82–86
　Terry Gray, 2, 54–57, 69
Peterson, Ronald, 190
pilgrimage trail, 140–45
positive self-talk, 63–65
positive thinking, 61, 191
　cases of, 61–62
　See also emotions
"possible selves," 81–82. *See also*
　Burns, Tammey
posture, 17, 23–24
　breathing and, 44

white blood cells, 26–27
will
    to move, xiii
    See also determination
Williamson, Linda, 122–25, 130
Woodbury, Nola, 17–19
Wordsworth, William, 99

writing. *See* Walking Logs

Yin-Yang Breath: Earth and Sky
    (breathing and focusing
    technique), 48–49, 73, 92,
    152, 174